Guidelines for Health Supervision III

American Academy of Pediatrics
DEDICATED TO THE HEALTH OF ALL CHILDREN™

Third Edition — 1997, updated 2002
Second Edition — 1988
First Edition — 1985

Library of Congress Control Number: 2002101272

ISBN 1-58110-088-4

MA0021

For additional copies, contact:

American Academy of Pediatrics
PO Box 747
141 Northwest Point Blvd
Elk Grove Village, IL 60009-0747

The recommendations in this publication do not indicate an exclusive course of treatment or serve as a standard of medical care. Variations, taking into account individual circumstances, may be appropriate.

Committee on Psychosocial Aspects
of Child and Family Health 1995–1996

Martin T. Stein, MD, Chairperson, 1992-1996
Mark L. Wolraich, MD, Chairperson, 1996-2000
Javier Aceves, MD
Heidi M. Feldman, PhD, MD
Joseph F. Hagan, Jr, MD
Barbara Howard, MD
Ellen C. Perrin, MD
Anthony J. Richtsmeier, MD
Deborah Tolchin, MD
Hyman C. Tolmas, MD

Liaison Representatives

F. Daniel Armstrong, PhD, Society of Pediatric Psychology
David R. DeMaso, MD, American Academy of Child and Adolescent Psychiatry
Rebecca Kajander, CPNP, MPH, National Association of Pediatric Nurse Associates and
    Practitioners
William J. Mahoney, MD, Canadian Paediatric Society

Consultants

George J. Cohen, MD, National Consortium for Child Mental Health Services
Conway Saylor, PhD, Society of Pediatric Psychology

Consultants to Revised Edition

George J. Cohen, MD
Joseph F. Hagan, Jr, MD (Chairperson, 2000-2002)

Staff

Karen Smith, Project Manager

Appreciation to:

The Committee gratefully acknowledges the assistance of the following individuals who also contributed to the development of this manual.

Past chairpersons of the Committee on Psychosocial Aspects of Child and Family Health contributed significantly to the first two editions of *Guidelines for Health Supervision:*
Drs Barbara Korsch, Morris Green, and Robert Pantell.

Natalie Arndt, Word Processor, Department of Maternal, Child and Adolescent Health, American Academy of Pediatrics

Barb Scotese, Senior Medical Copy Editor, Department of Maternal, Child and Adolescent Health, American Academy of Pediatrics

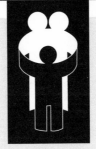

Table of Contents

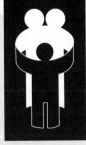

Preface

The supervision of health care during infancy, childhood, and adolescence is a complex process with many competing agendas in the areas of biomedical, developmental, and psychosocial aspects of pediatric practice. In recent years, the American Academy of Pediatrics (AAP) has provided a framework to help clinicians focus on important issues at developmentally appropriate time intervals. *Guidelines for Health Supervision,* now in its third edition, provides selected, focused approaches to caring for children and families whose health and adaptation are thought to be in the normal range. These approaches incorporate biomedical, developmental, and psychosocial information and are intended to be flexible, with the final agenda for health supervision determined principally by the relationship between practitioners and family members as well as by the needs and resources of individual children and their parents. The frequency, timing, and length of visits and health care priorities need to be individualized (see Appendix A, Recommendations for Preventive Pediatric Health Care). When appropriate, health care supervision can be shared among several health professionals. Educational resources (such as printed brochures, instructions, and audiovisual materials) offered in the setting of — *but not instead of* — doctor-patient interaction also contribute to comprehensive child health supervision.

One of the many benefits from comprehensive health supervision over time is the opportunity for practitioners to know the child and other family members well. This kind of relationship encourages families to turn more readily to their pediatrician for help with unexpected problems and stresses.

To prepare *Guidelines for Health Supervision III,* the AAP conducted an extensive systematic review of the second edition. Practitioners, academicians, and other experts provided many suggestions to assist in the task of revising the manual. We are grateful for the many thoughtful reviews from a variety of AAP committee members and practitioners. The main content of the *Guidelines,* because it was found useful by most practitioners, has not been changed. As anticipated, some practitioners found that the material was well known to them from their experience and education. A considerable amount of basic information has been retained, however, since these *Guidelines* are being used extensively in teaching programs for physicians and other health professionals. Each chapter, to be complete, contains some duplication and repetition of information. Cue cards summarizing this information are provided for convenient reference.

The therapeutic alliance between pediatricians and their patients and families is the context in which all other features of child health supervision, counseling, and guidance take place. The following chapter describes this important alliance. Specific suggestions for interview questions are given throughout this edition.

Direct communication with the child is emphasized because of the mounting evidence that more active participation by the child, even during the preschool years, enhances the doctor-patient relationship, enriches the information obtained by the physician, and has beneficial effects on the child's own health behavior. The current edition of the *Guidelines* encourages the clinician to seek information from the child and parent simultaneously.

Traditional areas of health supervision are addressed in the *Guidelines,* such as the detection of physical abnormalities accessible to intervention, preventive medicine, immunization against preventable diseases, nutrition, accident prevention, and emergency care. Many of these topics are discussed in further detail in other AAP publications. Explicit attention is given to monitoring child development; to observing interactions between the parent and child, parent and physician, and child and physician; and to exploring family interactions, including those that develop following a divorce, in single-parent families, and in families in which both parents work outside of the home.

The *Guidelines* incorporate suggestions for determining and promoting the strengths and potential resources of families and their individual members. Because self-esteem, confidence, and a sense of competence are essential for optimal adaptation and cooperation in health care, particular approaches to history taking, anticipatory guidance, and counseling are suggested to support, acknowledge, and reinforce independence and active participation by the child and family.

Supplemental information provided at the end of these *Guidelines* elaborates on some important developmental and psychosocial issues, such as sleep disorders, temper tantrums, problems in family life and child rearing practices, individual differences, and the development of a child with a challenging temperament. These supplements assist the pediatrician with common problems within the normal range of behavior and family relationships. For more complex situations requiring counseling and specially scheduled conference visits with the pediatrician, guidelines are available from AAP policy statements and selected references (see Appendix B, American Academy of Pediatrics Publications for Pediatricians and Parents and Other Caregivers).

The primary goal of this publication is to assist pediatric practitioners to promote optimal health and well-being of patients and their families. This function has become increasingly important as concerns over the cost of health care are modifying the nature of medical practice. By defining the scope of comprehensive pediatric care more clearly, we hope also to encourage research on the process, outcomes, costs, and benefits of this care.

Establishing a Therapeutic Alliance

Introduction

It is important that pediatricians engage patients and families as partners in support of their self-esteem, confidence, and competence. This goal can be achieved best in the context of personal and family centered care, continuity and accessibility of care, and sensitive interviewing that focuses on the strengths and values of children and their families. Optimally effective health care is based on active collaboration between families and health care professionals according to the family's expectations and main concerns and their readiness for new knowledge and advice.

Potential of the Therapeutic Alliance

When pediatricians succeed in engaging parents and children as partners in the supervision of health care, the task becomes easier and health care is more effective. The powerful therapeutic potential of the interactions of pediatricians with families is not always sufficiently realized. In order to achieve the most effective working relationship (or, more technically the ideal "therapeutic alliance") with patients, pediatricians must be responsive consistently to contributions of children and parents while being aware of their own resources and limitations (Table 1). Effective cooperation among physician, family, and associated health professionals is needed to achieve optimal function and adaptation for the child and family, both biologically and socially.

Impact Beyond Actual Encounters

Actual time spent by pediatricians with their patients, even in the first year of life, is limited; however, if the pediatrician gives parents and other caregivers access to appropriate health information and boosts their self-esteem, the impact may extend to the family's care of the child 24 hours a day, 365 days per year. There is increasing evidence that regardless of the specific health knowledge they profess, patients with low self-confidence and self-esteem are less motivated to engage in appropriate health care behaviors, such as preventive measures and prescribed medical regimens. An egalitarian, respectful approach to the patient as a partner in health care promotes self-esteem and self-confidence.

Physician Effectiveness

The quality of the physician's relationship with the patient can have a significant impact on the patient's competence, sense of confidence, health attitudes, and behavior. Physicians are endowed with tremendous credibility by both patients and society. Patients visit their physicians for help with specific needs and concerns, wanting reassurance, information, and advice. Since patients often are anxious when they consult a physician, their feelings of vulnerability and anxiety result in varying levels of readiness for accepting the information that is offered.

A number of features of the pediatrician's practice can enhance the therapeutic potential. A continuing relationship with the family begins with the prenatal visit and extends to the examination immediately after the infant's birth in the hospital. Patterns for future health care with the parents can be established at these visits. Optimal opportunities also exist at these visits for interweaving the biologic and psychosocial aspects of care.

Table 1.

Physician Strategies for Enhancing Therapeutic Potential
• Continued comprehensive, personalized, family-centered approach
• Realistic recognition of limitations in self, patient, time, and environment
• Effectively planned use of time
• Respect for patients' agendas and solutions
• Communication of trust and respect; sensitive awareness of patients' needs expectations, and concerns, as well as their resources and limitations

Pediatricians play many roles, including teacher, helper, counselor, and healer. The action-oriented pediatrician who focuses on diagnosis and treatment may find the role of "listener" difficult. It is important to remember that many patients and parents need and appreciate a well-informed, skilled, nonjudgmental person who listens respectfully to their concerns.

Receptiveness of Parents

Parents of young children are open to professional expert advice. Single parents, mothers who work outside the home, parents who are emotionally immature, and parents who are ambivalent about childbearing and parenting are especially vulnerable to feelings of self-blame, guilt, and anxiety. The pediatrician who recognizes the potential for good parenting and cooperation in these vulnerable parents can be a source of tremendous strength and support. A dogmatic, authoritarian, patronizing pediatrician may risk having the opposite effect. Comments such as, "You came to me just in time," make parents more anxious and dependent. On the other hand, an encouraging remark such as, "You are really taking good care of your son during these difficult times," reinforces parental confidence and enhances performance.

Physician-Patient Communication Process

Eric Cassell writes that physicians should be as careful in their use of words as in their prescription of drugs. It is largely in the use of language during the process of reasoned doctor-patient communication that the physician realizes therapeutic potential. Nonjudgmental, open-ended interview techniques that facilitate participation in health care by parents and patients need not lead to inappropriately lengthy or costly interactions. Evidence suggests quite the opposite; namely, facilitation of communication helps pediatricians and patients to accomplish their common tasks more expeditiously (Table 2). However, patients and parents who feel unheard and poorly understood are frustrated in their attempts to engage the pediatrician's attention and may persevere in time-consuming efforts to express their concerns.

Careful, objective observation of parent-child interaction while the child is being examined and during procedures provides valuable information for the physician. A few words directed toward the patient's caregiver (mother, father, grandmother) as a person with needs, feelings, and interests are received enthusiastically and make the interaction more rewarding for all concerned. Including family members and other important persons in the interaction provides the basis for a rewarding relationship and future cooperation. Common courtesies are essential, such as knocking before entering examining rooms, greeting children directly, addressing patients by their preferred names, dressing appropriately, protecting the privacy of patients, and minimizing interruptions. Appropriate boundaries between pediatricians and patients and between

Table 2.

Communication Skills in Pediatrician-Family Interaction

Goal	Example
Boost self-esteem.	"You're doing a great job."
Enhance sense of confidence and competence.	
Consider the patient and family as the partners in problem solving.	"How can I help you deal with the problem?"
Be open-ended.	"Tell me about Billy."
Be nonjudgmental.	"In this situation, anyone would get impatient."
Respect the family's agenda and timetable.	"What concerns you the most about Cathy at this time?"
Explore the family's value system.	"Have you discussed this problem with anyone else (your priest, etc)?"
Use family's own resources and approaches.	"Tell me what you've tried up to now. What seemed to work best?"
Make advice finite, practical, and concrete.	"Do you think you could listen to him cry for about 10 minutes before going to pick him up?"
Allow yourself time to enjoy the patient as a person.	"What is your favorite time at school — class time or recess?"
Make "contract" explicit.	"How would you like to spend the time we have left before the end of our appointment?"
Don't underrate your own therapeutic potential.	"This must be a really tough time for you; your next appointment is in 2 weeks, but please call me on Wednesday and let me know how things are going."

pediatricians and their patients' parents are the responsibility of the pediatrician. Behavior and communication that could be interpreted as having romantic or sexual meaning must be avoided. Acceptance of gifts or other nonmonetary compensation for medical services is not recommended.

Encouragement for parents and children to participate actively in the visit is helpful. Examples include: "We have 5 more minutes; would you like to spend them discussing the discipline problem you mentioned earlier?" "What else would you like to concentrate on today?" "You seem to be upset with some of the questions I asked you today." "What I have just told you seems to make you angry; I am curious to know why." "You don't seem too hopeful that what I have suggested will work; will you help me understand why?" "You seem very worried about _____ today."

Before possible solutions are offered in response to patient questions or concerns, it is crucial to inquire what approaches the patient and family have already tried, have thought of doing, or are planning to do so that their own efforts are not dismissed. The family's own solution may be more likely to succeed because it arises within their value system and thus encourages independence and resourcefulness.

When sensitive interviewing and listening by the pediatrician bring to light psychosocial or other problems that require time commitments beyond the anticipated office visit, a separate, longer "conference" appointment should be scheduled. If the problem seems beyond the scope of the pediatrician's confidence or interest, the patient should be referred promptly to a professional in a related discipline (social work, psychology, or psychiatry, for example). Treatment received from another professional will be more effective if the pediatrician remains actively supportive.

Communication With the Child

During the pediatric visit, the child's role deserves separate attention. All discussion in the child's presence must be planned with full awareness of the child's feelings and level of understanding.

Young infants respond to many elements of an examiner's voice as well as to touch and other behaviors. Consequently, an appropriate tone of voice, secure setting (on a parent's lap), warm examining hands, and a bright toy may be helpful. Toddlers can be especially difficult to approach and are least likely to respond to the pediatrician's friendly demeanor or a colorful distracter.

By the time children are 3 years old, they are curious and cautious and can generally be engaged in conversation about colors, names, and toys. Although they may fluctuate from magical to concrete thinking, concepts about health and illness begin to have meaning. Statements such as "your heart is strong" and "you're not sick now" are understandable and may please and reassure the child.

Conversation during examinations with school-age children becomes easier, and a considerable amount of information about health and illness can be gathered and imparted directly. This exchange of information also can demonstrate to children their important contribution to staying healthy and recovering from illness. This topic is expanded in the prefaces of the sections on school-age years and adolescence.

When highly charged discussions about behavior occur when the child is present, the physician can include the child in the discussion, eg, "Your mom gets pretty angry with you when you take things off the shelves in the market, doesn't she? How do you feel about that?" or "Do you think you could stop nagging your mom to buy you candy if you could earn a treat by doing something special to help her in the house?" The pediatrician can also reassure the child by addressing the mother, eg, "I can understand how angry you get when he does that — any mother would — but remember how proud you were during the last visit when you told me how well he feeds and dresses himself?"

Magical Expectations From Physicians

The physician's word often becomes a family truth. Children and parents may have unrealistic expectations, looking to physicians for magic, wisdom, and cures. Physicians may be regarded with both admiration and fear. In their privileged role, they are allowed to break taboos, to hear secrets, to touch private parts of the body, to look into orifices, to stick needles, and to hurt.

Physicians have very high expectations of themselves — faultless performance, superior technical skills, high levels of compassion and patience, and access to an up-to-date database. Some believe that it is unreasonable to be expected also to fine tune the doctor-patient interaction and remain sensitive and responsive to patients' interpersonal needs. Certainly under stress practitioners may fall short of what they perceive as ideal. They sometimes lose their tempers, get angry, fail to pick up on patient cues, hurry through visits, or make tactless remarks. Even from this standpoint, establishing a therapeutic alliance is an important safeguard. By presenting themselves as less God-like and omnipotent, pediatricians prepare the family for their imperfections. In the presence of a warm relationship, patient and physician tend to forgive each other's shortcomings. Also, in an established therapeutic alliance, the burdens are shared and easier to endure. Decisions are made jointly, procedures are planned cooperatively, doubts and fears are discussed, and miracles are no longer expected.

It would be simplistic to suggest that egalitarian relationships are best at all times for every patient and family. Patients also need the physicians' authoritative, informed decisions and counsel. There are times when patients are not ready to hear the whole truth, and there are times when they may need a little more reassurance than the facts warrant. There are also times when physicians are seen as omnipotent and given more credit than may be deserved. The physicians will pay for these instances by being blamed when blameless or criticized when doing well — it all evens out. Physicians who have developed a reasonable awareness of their own reactions can deal with these instances without overreacting or feeling unduly challenged, and without blaming or shaming their patients.

The tremendous therapeutic potential of the relationship between pediatricians, children, and their families often is not fully recognized. Full awareness of this potential serves to enhance both the effectiveness of pediatric practice and patients' and physicians' satisfaction in their relationship.

Suggested Readings

Cassell EJ. *The Healer's Art.* Cambridge, MA: MIT Press; 1976

Dixon SD, Stein MT. *Encounters With Children — Pediatric Behavior and Development.* St Louis, MO: Mosby-Year Book; 1992

Francis V, Korsch BM, Morris MJ. Gaps in doctor-patient communications: patients' response to medical advice. *N Engl J Med.* 1969;280:535–540

Green M. The pediatric interview and history. In: Green M, Haggerty RJ, eds. *Ambulatory Pediatrics Four.* Philadelphia, PA: WB Saunders Co; 1990:578–581

Korsch BM, Negrete VF. Doctor-patient communication. *Sci Am.* 1972; 227:66–74

Lipkin MR, Putnam SM, Lazare A. *The Medical Interview: Clinical Care, Education, Research.* New York, NY: Springer Verlag; 1995

Platt, FW. *Conversation Repair.* Boston, MA: Little, Brown, & Co; 1995

Prugh DG. *The Psychosocial Aspects of Pediatrics.* Philadelphia, PA: Lea and Febiger; 1983:207–234

Responding to infants and parents. *Zero to Three.* February/March 2000;20:5–7

Encouraging Active Participation by Parents and Children in Child Health Supervision

In the process of revising the *Guidelines for Health Supervision,* the Committee created a set of parallel guidelines for parents (see Appendix C, Parent and Child Guides to Pediatric Visits). These guidelines are intended to help parents make systematic observations, to formulate their questions, and to communicate their concerns effectively to their pediatrician. The parent Guides were developed for six broad age categories. They may be completed at home or in the waiting area prior to a child's appointment. Each Guide consists of a short description of a particular age group and a set of questions to guide the observations and questions of parents. For older children, there are also child Guides.

These Guides are available to be distributed to parents and children by pediatricians, nurse practitioners, or office staff (see Appendix B, American Academy of Pediatrics Publications for Pediatricians and Parents and Other Caregivers). We anticipate that their use will enable pediatricians, parents, and children to communicate more effectively about child development, behavior, and family circumstances.

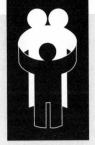

Health Supervision: The Prenatal Visit

Prenatal contact generally starts with a telephone call from a prospective parent to the physician's office asking about hours, fees, hospital affiliation, types of health insurance accepted, and emergency coverage; these questions may be answered by the staff or by the physician. This contact establishes an initial relationship between the office staff and a parent. During this conversation, the parent should be invited to schedule a prenatal visit with the pediatric clinician, including both parents, if possible.

A visit is recommended for all expectant families. It is especially valuable for first pregnancies; parents new to the practice; single parents; families with high-risk pregnancies, pregnancy complications, or multiple gestation; and parents who have previously experienced a perinatal death. This visit may also be valuable to parents planning to adopt a child.

The chief objectives of the visit are as follows: (1) to establish a good working relationship with the family before the birth of their child, (2) to assess perinatal risk factors, (3) to provide anticipatory guidance regarding infant care and family adjustment, (4) to perform a psychosocial assessment of the family, (5) to introduce the health care providers and prepare parents for the availability and utilization of primary care services, (6) to provide an opportunity for parents to ask questions, (7) to discuss plans for feeding the infant, and (8) to respond to questions about circumcision. The pediatrician helps the parents feel comfortable about expressing their anxieties, concerns, and expectations about the pregnancy and new baby. A thoughtful approach to questions permits the mutual assessment and clarification necessary for personalized pediatric care.

Gathering Information/Anticipatory Guidance

Some parents will ask questions readily, whereas others will appreciate being given the basic information needed. The use of a printed questionnaire that parents could complete in the waiting room before the interview may suggest issues that should be emphasized during the visit. Advice provided to families should be individualized to their beliefs, values, experiences, and needs. To facilitate family responsiveness, issues should be discussed fully with both parents and advice interwoven with the discussion. Whenever possible, families should be encouraged to participate actively in the decision-making process.

Some of the major issues to discuss are as follows:

◆ **Pregnancy**

How did you feel when you learned you were pregnant? How has your pregnancy gone? Have you experienced any illness? Taking medication? Does either of you smoke cigarettes, drink alcohol, or use illicit drugs?

Discuss the effects of using illicit drugs and medication on pregnancy.

❖ *Urge prospective mothers to stop smoking and to stop drinking alcohol and using illicit drugs during pregnancy.*

❖ *Urge other adults in the household or family to discontinue smoking or smoke outside the home because of the respiratory problems caused by passive smoke.*

◆ **Family and social history**

Who are the people in your families? Are there others living in your household? Are your family members healthy? What is your marital status, educational background, and occupation? Do any conditions run in your families (eg, anemia, sickle cell disease or trait, allergies, asthma, elevated cholesterol levels, excessive bleeding or bruising [especially if circumcision is planned], alcohol or other drug problems, hypertension, coronary heart disease, mental illness, convulsions, and any other diseases or conditions)? Is there a member of either family who had a baby with serious problems as a newborn? Are there pets in the house? Were previous pregnancies and deliveries uneventful? Who is available when you need support? What are your plans after the birth — returning to work outside the home or school? What are your child care arrangements?

◆ **Labor, delivery, and hospital stay**

What do you expect during labor and delivery? How have you prepared? What adults will be involved? How do you feel about rooming-in? How did things go after the birth of your other children? Any problems? Postpartum depression?

Urge participation in prenatal classes, if these are available in the community and if time before delivery permits. Encourage the active participation of the father or partner throughout the pregnancy and birth process. Otherwise consider other supportive family members or friends who can be present. Discuss the option of rooming-in, if it is available. Discuss plans for the return home from the hospital by securing help with household chores and the care of the baby's siblings. Mothers with a history of postpartum depression are at risk for recurrence of depression with subsequent pregnancies and at other times.

◆ Nutrition

What are your plans for feeding the infant? Breastfeeding? Bottle-feeding? How much do you know about these methods of feeding?

The decision to breastfeed or bottle-feed is best made before delivery. For parents who have not decided on the method of feeding, discuss both approaches. A strong endorsement for breastfeeding should be made while supporting the parents' decision. For prospective mothers who plan to breastfeed, discuss how they can prepare for breastfeeding.* Inform the mother who plans to breastfeed that nursing a newborn is an "adult learning experience." It may come naturally, but more often requires learning about holding techniques, latching-on behaviors of the baby, and the infant's sucking process. By the third day of life, when most babies discover that their mother's milk is plentiful, nursing is usually well established. Let them know that they will receive help with breastfeeding in the hospital. The availability of a lactation consultant and office-based support after hospital discharge for women who breastfeed should be emphasized. Recommendations of the type and quantity of formula should be provided to parents who plan to bottle-feed. Also discuss family history of milk allergy/intolerance.

◆ Circumcision

If you have a boy, what are your plans regarding circumcision?

The decision about circumcision is best made prenatally. Discuss the potential risks and benefits of this procedure. Family preference should be determined and supported.

◆ Sleeping arrangements

Where will your infant sleep? What type of crib or other furniture do you have?

Advise parents about crib safety. Slats should be less than $2\frac{3}{8}$ inches apart. Mattress and its covering should be snug-fitting. Avoid quilts, sheepskin, or other soft surfaces. Pillows and stuffed animals should not be in the infant's sleeping environment. Newborns should sleep face up. Avoid overheating the infant. Advise parents about the potential hazards of cosleeping.

---

*See the AAP brochure, "A Woman's Guide to Beastfeeding," available from the AAP.

◆ Child rearing

What have you learned about baby care from reading, from friends/ family, from baby-sitting as a youth? Have you attended prenatal classes? If so, how much time was dedicated to child care issues? How will having a baby change your lives? How do you plan to rear your baby? How is your plan different from how you were raised?

Written materials on infant care are very useful and may be recommended.*

◆ Social relationships

What do you think the impact of the new baby will be on your other children? What extended family members or friends will be available to help you care for your baby? Explore cultural attributes that may affect child care.

Prepare for potential changes in family relationships upon the baby's birth.

Discuss the need to balance roles as parents with those learned as a couple.

Review the needs of siblings

❖ *Discuss ways to involve older children in preparing for the new baby.*

❖ *Review arrangements for their care during the mother's hospital stay.*

❖ *Advise parents to prepare their children for separation from their mother while she is in the hospital.*

❖ *Discuss the possibility that toddlers may regress in some skills that were already achieved (eg, using the toilet).*

❖ *Discuss hospital rules for sibling visitation.*

◆ Safety Issues

Stress the importance of car safety restraints. Advise parents to have the car seat for their infant ready for the ride home from the hospital.†

Discuss home safety. Impress upon parents the importance of having smoke detectors, a fire extinguisher, and an escape plan. Advise them about safe behaviors during fires, initial burn treatment, and adequate supervision of children in order to prevent fires. The maximum water heater temperature should be set at 120°F to avoid accidental scalding.

Suggest that parents learn CPR for infants and children.

---

*See the AAP book, *Caring for Your Baby and Young Child. Birth to Age 5*, available from the AAP.

†See the AAP brochure, "2001 Family Shopping Guide to Car Seats," available from the AAP.

Stress the importance of not smoking. Inform parents of the relationship of environmental tobacco smoke to respiratory illness, SIDS (sudden infant death syndrome), middle ear effusions, and cancer in adulthood. Suggest strategies for smoking cessation. Advise parents about violence prevention.

◆ **Pediatric care**

Provide a listing of all other professional staff: other pediatricians, nurse practitioners, office nurses. Review how parents can schedule visits and receive unscheduled or emergency care. Inform parents about which hospital to use for an emergency situation. Review the office hours and office telephone triage system. Describe the format for health supervision visits with an emphasis on developmental surveillance and the opportunity to raise concerns or ask questions. Describe the immunization schedule (see the current Recommended Childhood Immunization Schedule). Discuss any special support services available through the office including breastfeeding counseling, social services, and parenting classes.

Closing the Visit

◆ Ask whether the parents have any other questions.

◆ Inform the parents how and when to notify the pediatrician at the time of the birth.

◆ Encourage the parents to telephone the office if questions or problems arise prior to delivery.

◆ Convey congratulations and best wishes to the parents.

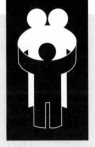

Health Supervision: Newborn Visit

The hospital visit should be performed within the first 24 hours of age. If the baby is staying in the hospital for more than 24 hours, visits should be performed every day or two (depending on the medical condition of the baby).

Introductions Between Parents and the Pediatrician

If a prenatal visit with the parents (one or both) has taken place, the bond that already exists with the family will be appreciated, creating an increased sense of enjoyment of the newborn. It also will be easier for the parents to ask questions about the baby.

If a prenatal visit has not taken place, and you haven't already met, introduce yourself and explain why you are seeing the baby, eg, "Dr Jones, the obstetrician who delivered you, asked me to check the baby," or "I am the doctor the hospital has seeing all the newborns today." Give the mother your card, or write your name down for her and explain how you can be reached.

Ask to be introduced to any visitors who might be with the parents.

Congratulate the parents and any siblings.

Ask if there are any questions or concerns about the baby.

Health Assessment

Interview

For the initial newborn visits in the hospital.

❖ *Review the notes and comments of the nurses.*

Welcoming questions

◆ How are you feeling? How are the baby's father and your other children? Have they visited?

◆ How is the baby feeding? Have you changed the baby's diaper yet? Was it wet? What was the bowel movement like? How do you feel handling the baby?

Physical Examination

It is a good idea to examine the newborn in the presence of the parents so you can point out any significant findings and be reassuring about any minor findings that may cause anxiety after the baby is taken home. Make sure to demonstrate the undressed infant in both the prone and supine positions. Observe how the parents relate to the baby. Do they appear competent and confident? How responsive are they to the newborn? Observe the relationship of the mother with significant others, such as the baby's father, grandmother, and other children.

Measurements: *measure and plot percentiles*

◆ Length

◆ Weight

◆ Head circumference

Perform a full examination

As part of the complete physical examination, assess gestational age, check the red reflex, palpate the clavicles, listen carefully for a heart murmur, examine for signs of hip dislocation or dislocatability, check the femoral pulses and the genitalia, evaluate movement of all four limbs, and survey neonatal reflexes. Assess jaundice if noted. Check the child's feet for clubfoot or metatarsus adductus. See that the newborn's hearing is tested using a physiologic screening method during the first 24 to 48 hours after birth.

Common findings that should be explained to the parents include salmon patches at the nape of the neck and face, puffy eyelids, subconjunctival hemorrhages, engorged breasts, mottling of skin, acrocyanosis, molding of the skull, cephalohematoma, Moro startle reaction, mongoloid spots, chin quivering, and erythema toxicum neonatorum. Pigmented nevi present at birth should be called to the attention of the parents.

Screening Procedures

Review the mother's laboratory information for relevant reports, eg, serologic test for syphilis; hepatitis B surface antigen, group B streptococcus, gonococcus, and chlamydia cervical screening tests; and human immunodeficiency virus antibody.

Check for evidence of blood incompatibility between the mother and baby.

Screen for phenylketonuria and other disorders (hypothyroidism, hemoglobinopathies, galactosernia) prior to discharge or after 24 hours of age according to state law.

Formulation and Plan

Health Maintenance

Immunizations

Hepatitis B (first dose) may be given during the newborn period.

Anticipatory guidance

◆ **Review feedings**
  Newborns should be fed on demand. If the newborn is breastfed, discuss the duration of each feeding, alternating breasts during feeding, and vitamin D supplementation, if indicated (in infants who are either dark skinned or who have limited sunlight exposure during the first year). Help the mother find the most comfortable nursing position. Nursing should be initiated as soon as the baby is stable and the mother is alert. Remind the mother to drink a lot of fluids. If the newborn is fed formula, discuss the type of formula that can be used. Bottles should not be warmed in the microwave. When the baby is fed, the bottle should be held, not propped.

◆ **Sleeping position and sleeping environment**
Advise that the baby be placed down for sleep in a supine position. A standard firm infant mattress with no more than a thin covering, such as a sheet or rubberized pad, should be used. Soft, plush, or bulky items, such as quilts, blankets, sheepskin, pillows, rolls of bedding, or cushions, should not be in the infant's immediate sleeping environment.

◆ **Care of the skin**
Sponge bathe the newborn until the umbilical cord falls off and the cord area looks normal. The base of the cord looks yellow and is slightly wet before and after the cord falls off; there may be some blood staining. Keep the area clean with alcohol until the cord is off and the area is dry. Bathe the baby daily; clean the diaper area with warm water after bowel movements.

◆ **Other care issues**
Newborn girls will have a vaginal mucus discharge, possibly with blood. This is a normal response to estrogen withdrawal similar to what the mother is experiencing and is not a cause for alarm. The rectal area in girls is cleaned from the front backwards so rectal germs are not brought forward to the urethra. All stool should be removed by cleansing with a mild soap and water; the vaginal discharge may be allowed to remain.

Newborn boys as well as newborn girls may have some breast engorgement at birth, which may become more severe over the next several weeks before resolving; this is normal, even with a colostrum-like secretion. Advise the parents not to try to reduce the swelling by expressing fluid from the nipples, which may cause infection.

If the newborn boy is to be circumcised, discuss care of the penis.

◆ **Family and other visitors**
Parents, grandparents, and siblings may have close contact with the newborn. Avoid close contact with nonhousehold members and especially avoid contact with anyone who has a cold or contagious condition. Visitors may tire the mother at a time when she is already exhausted from the labor and delivery and getting little sleep; suggest to the mother that friends and relatives do chores and errands for her and that social visits can be limited for the first few weeks.

◆ **Safety practices**
The baby should never be left in the direct rays of the sun because the skin could burn. The baby may be taken outside if properly dressed for the temperature.

To prevent falls, the baby should never be left alone on the bed, changing table, or in the crib with the side down.

Crib slats should be less than $2\frac{3}{8}$ inches apart.

Crib bumpers should be used.

Toys with long strings and pacifiers that hang from a string around the baby's neck must be avoided.

The baby should not be left alone with young siblings or pets.

The water heater thermostat needs to be set at 120°F to avoid accidental scalding.

Smoke detectors should be installed and maintained in their home.

Infants, when riding in a car, must always be properly belted into a car seat that is properly affixed. Determine that parents have accurate information about car safety seats and their proper installation and that they have a proper car safety seat. Advise parents who drive a pickup truck about the appropriate safety seat for the vehicle.

Infants should sleep face up on their back.

A tobacco-free and drug-free environment is important.

Suggest that parents learn CPR for infants and children.

Advise parents about violence prevention.

◆ **Recognition of illness**
The physician must be notified if the skin or the whites of the infant's eyes appear yellow; a prompt blood test may be necessary.

Parents need to have a thermometer and know how to take the baby's temperature if they are concerned that the baby may be sick. The physician should be called if the newborn has a fever, refuses to feed, vomits persistently, has diarrhea, is unusually irritable or somnolent, or just does not look well.

◆ **Supporting the family**
Encourage closeness with the baby, eg, holding, rocking, fondling, talking.

Remind the parents that their baby is unique. A wide range of normal behavior exists for crying and sleeping (some newborns may cry as much as 2 to 3 hours a day and cry 10 to 15 minutes before falling asleep; sleep may vary between 12 and 20 hours a day). The infant should be placed in the crib awake (see supplement on Sleep Problems, p 219).

Parents should encourage and support each other in the care of the newborn.

The siblings should be encouraged to participate in closely supervised care of the newborn, eg, "Get me a diaper," "Let me know if he is awake," or "Pat him on his hand like this." Also, stress to each sibling his or her specialness in the family. Encourage the parents to set aside time for each older sibling when the baby is sleeping or in the care of someone else.

The next few weeks will be exciting and wonderful, but will also be stressful and tiring. Encourage the mother to plan rest periods. Advise her to call her physician if she experiences postpartum "blues."

Problems and Plans

List each problem identified with a plan of management.

Closing the Visit

◆ **Restate your impression of the baby, eg, "He is doing fine," or "He is stable but we are keeping an eye on his breathing."**

◆ **Compliment the parents on their ability to comfort the infant, to ask intelligent questions, and to be mutually supportive. Also mention the infant's developmental strengths, eg, how responsive he (or she) is to the parent.**

◆ **Discharge planning.**
Is the home prepared for the newborn? Are the siblings (if any) prepared for the newborn? Who will help the mother at home? Are any difficulties anticipated in getting the baby into the office for follow-up visits?

◆ **Ask if there are any other concerns that need to be discussed. Suggest that the parents write down questions as they occur to them so they can be answered at the next bedside, telephone, or office contact.**

◆ **Discuss the next contact with the family.**
If the baby remains in the hospital, inform the parents of when follow-up visits will occur.

If the baby is being discharged, advise the parents when and how the first office visit should be scheduled.

Premature babies, infants of mothers who are teenagers or who have mental health problems, or other infants at high risk should be seen within a week.

If the infant is being discharged in less than 24 hours, an examination within 48 hours of discharge should be arranged either by a home nursing visit or an office appointment. You may want to see the infant within a couple of days (see supplement on Parental Stress and the Child at Risk, p 233).

Inform parents about which hospital to use for an emergency situation. Make sure the parents know how to contact the office should they have any questions or worries.

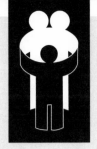

Health Supervision: 2- to 4-Week-Old Visit

Health Assessment

Infants at this young age feed frequently. Their sleep cycle may be erratic. They are totally dependent on adults for care and comfort. Parents may be quite tired because of the high demands of care and the lack of uninterrupted sleep. The first office visit is the opportunity to assess the adjustment of both child and family.

Interview With Behavioral Observations

Throughout the interview observe the emotional state of the parents or caregivers. Do they seem pleased and comfortable with the baby, or overwhelmed, or depressed? Pay attention to how the parents interact with their infant and with each other.

Welcoming questions

How are you? How is the baby? What issues or concerns do you want to discuss at this visit?

Check on the status of any issues addressed at the prenatal and/or newborn visit.

Specific questions about the infant

- ◆ **Review the birth history including birth weight, gestational age, problems.**

◆ **Nutrition**

Is the infant breastfed or bottle-fed (type of formula)? Review frequency, duration, and amount of feedings. Is the infant receiving vitamins, fluoride?

◆ **Elimination**

During elimination of stool or urine, does the infant seem distressed? How often does the infant urinate? How often does he or she have a bowel movement? Describe the pattern of the urinary stream (in males).

◆ **Sleep patterns**

How long does the baby sleep at a stretch? How many hours out of 24 does the baby sleep? Do you hold or rock the baby to sleep or do you put the baby into the crib while awake? How do you put the baby to bed?

◆ **Behavior and development**

Can your infant raise his or her head slightly when lying prone? When the infant is in a quiet-alert state, does he or she: Blink in reaction to bright light? Fixate on a face or object and follow movement? Startle in reaction to a loud noise? How do you tell what your infant wants or needs? Can you tell by the cry?

When your infant becomes fussy or upset, what do you do that calms him or her?

How has the infant changed since birth? Ask the parents to describe the infant's personality.

Questions about the family

How are you managing caring for the baby? How has it affected your sleep? Who is available to help you at home? What do you do when things seem to be getting to you? How are your other children doing?

What are each parent's plans now about working outside the home? Who will care for the baby if both parents are working?

Inquire about smoking, pets, and recent family stresses.

◆ **Completion of the family history**

If a complete family history was not recorded at the prenatal visit or when the infant was in the nursery, ask about the age, occupation, and health history of the parents and other members of the household. Confirm that the mother is rubella-immune. Determine any illnesses in the family that may be inheritable. Inquire about family background of:

❖ *anemia, including sickle cell and thalassemia*

❖ *heart disease*

❖ *cholesterol problems*

❖ *excessive bleeding or bruising*

❖ *emotional problems*

❖ *problems with drinking or drugs*

❖ *history of violence or abuse*

Physical Examination With Behavioral Observations

Observe the confidence and competence of the parents in handling the baby; observe infant-caregiver interactions.

Measurements: *measure and plot percentiles*

◆ Height

◆ Weight

◆ Head circumference

◆ The infant should be weighed undressed or wearing only a diaper.

General physical examination

To keep the infant as comfortable as possible, perform the least invasive procedures first: use your eyes, then your hands, then your instruments. Your stethoscope is less invasive than your otoscope.

As part of the complete physical examination, make sure to check the infant's red reflex, listen carefully for cardiac murmurs, and examine for abdominal masses and hip dislocation. Assess hearing.

Observe developmental progress (see Box, Typical Developmental Progress at 2 to 4 Weeks)

Screening Procedures

Review the results of newborn metabolic screening. Tests and reporting arrangements vary by state.

Typical Developmental Progress at 2 to 4 Weeks

- Raises head slightly from prone position
- Blinks in reaction to bright light
- Focuses and follows with eyes
- Responds to sound either by quieting or turning toward the source

Formulation and Plan

Strengths of the Family and Infant

Make positive statements about the baby's development and personality (eg, weight gain, alertness, responsiveness, ability to lift and turn head, muscle tone).

Acknowledge the parents' caregiving strengths, such as their observational skills and their ability to elicit a response from the baby.

Health Maintenance

Immunizations

Administer the second dose of hepatitis B vaccine at 1 month of age if the first dose was given at birth; administer the first dose if it was not given at birth.

Inform the parents that the diphtheria, tetanus, and pertussis (DTaP or DTP; DTaP is preferred; see Recommended Childhood Immunization Schedule, Appendix D), *Haemophilus influenzae* type b, and inactive poliovirus vaccines need to be given at the next health maintenance visit; give parents the Vaccine Information Statements.* The use of oral poliovirus vaccine (OPV) is not recommended except in special circumstances; if use of OPV is necessary, remind parents that immunosuppressed persons should not be in direct contact with an infant after immunization with OPV vaccine.

See the current Recommended Childhood Immunization Schedule.

*Vaccine Information Statements can be obtained from the AAP.

28

Anticipatory guidance

◆ Nutrition

Breastfeeding
Discuss potential difficulties with breastfeeding (inadequate milk available, sore nipples, or maternal fatigue).

Encourage adequate maternal diet and fluid intake.

Formula
Inform the parents to feed the baby only until the baby is satisfied; the baby does not need to finish each bottle.

Advise parents not to heat bottles in the microwave.

Solid foods
Solid foods should not be added to the diet at this time and may be started between 4 and 6 months of age unless specifically contraindicated.

Vitamins
Consider administering vitamin D (400 IU/d) to breastfed infants who are either dark skinned or who have limited sunlight exposure.

Provide fluoride supplementation to the infant if the water supply is not fluoridated.

◆ Elimination

Explain normal variations in stool frequency, color, and consistency. The urine stream of boys should be straight and forceful.

◆ Sleep patterns

Suggest that night feedings be shared between the parents or between the mother and another caregiver so that the mother can get sufficient sleep. Although the father cannot share breastfeeding he can participate in feeding by activities such as bringing the baby to mother and changing the diaper. Suggest that the parent(s) nap during the day while the baby sleeps. Explain techniques for altering the position of the baby in the crib to avoid excessive flat areas on the occiput.

◆ Development and behavior

Over the next month it is likely that the baby's schedule will become more regular, and he or she will become more sociable. This is a good age to make or obtain a mobile, since babies begin fixing their vision on moving and bright-colored objects, and a rattle because babies start to grasp and hold onto objects. Encourage parents to place their baby in a prone position occasionally while awake.

Parents should be encouraged to talk to babies to stimulate language development; over the next month the baby can be expected to start cooing and attending with interest when someone talks or sings to him or her.

Crying, especially in the late afternoon and early evening, may increase during the first 6 to 8 weeks; 2 to 3 hours of crying a day is normal in the first 3 months. If the baby is crying, the parents should check the diaper and consider whether the baby may be hungry. More often, a physical reason for crying cannot be found. Parents generally learn by experience when to pick up and console the baby and when to feel confident that the infant will stop crying alone in a few minutes. Responding to their infant's crying will not result in the infant being "spoiled" or overcoddled. Parents should call the pediatrician if the baby's persistent crying becomes very upsetting.

A comprehensive evaluation is indicated in infants who do not respond to sound or who have abnormally increased or decreased muscle tone.

◆ Social/family relationships

Encourage the mother or primary caregiver to arrange for a few hours of personal time during each week.

Encourage the parents to spend time together as well as to maintain their family and social relationships and activities. Explore the needs for additional support from extended family, friends, or parent groups.

Review the need to provide additional attention for each of the other children.

Mention "baby blues."

◆ Injury prevention

Infants should never be left alone in the car. Infants must be secured in car seats; parents should wear seat belts.

Smoke detectors are essential in the home.

Hot water heaters should be set at 120°F to avoid accidental scalding.

The newborn should sleep on his or her back and soft, porous sleeping surfaces should be avoided.

The baby should never be left unattended on a dressing table, bed, or couch. Pillows used as barriers around the baby will not prevent a fall.

A washcloth under the baby may diminish slipping in the bathtub.

Strings should not be used to tie pacifiers, toys, or medallions around the baby's neck or around the slats of the crib.

Advise parents never to shake their baby.

Guns in the home are a danger to the family. If a gun is kept in the home, advise parents to store the gun and ammunition in locked, separate locations. (Pediatricians and other child health care professionals are urged to inform parents about the dangers of guns in and outside the home. The AAP recommends that pediatricians incorporate questions about guns into their patient history taking and urge parents who possess guns to remove them, especially handguns, from the home.) Also advise parents about other strategies for violence prevention.

Emphasize the importance of a tobacco-free and drug-free environment.

Advise parents about protection from UV light.

Problems and Plans

Review other issues and plans to address them.

Closing the Visit

◆ **Were your goals for this visit met? Are there other issues you want to discuss? New concerns raised at this point may require scheduling a visit sooner than the next routine visit.**

◆ **Set a time for the next appointment.**

◆ **Indicate how to contact the office should any concerns arise prior to the next scheduled visit.**

◆ **Call earlier than next scheduled visit if the child is ill, crying does not subside and seems hard to manage, or parents feel unable to care for the infant adequately.**

◆ **Review with parents the procedures for emergency and nonroutine office visits.**

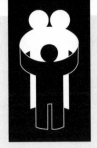

Health Supervision: 2-Month-Old Visit

Health Assessment

Most 2-month-old babies have already become responsive to their parents by smiling, cooing, and vocalizing reciprocally with them. While babies by this age may have established a regular schedule of feedings and sleeping, they are still very demanding and require a great deal of attention from their parents. Maternal depression persisting to this time is a serious clinical concern.

Interview With Behavioral Observations

Throughout the interview and physical examination, observe the parents' interactions with the infant.

Welcoming questions

How is your baby? How are you? What issues or concerns do you want to discuss at this visit?

Check on the status of issues discussed at the previous visit.

Specific questions about the infant

◆ Nutrition

Do you have any questions or concerns about breastfeeding? How often and how long does the baby feed? Are you giving the baby supplements of formula, water, vitamins, and/or fluoride? If the parents are bottle-feeding the infant, ask how many ounces the baby drinks during a feeding. How frequent are the feedings?

◆ Elimination

How many soiled diapers do you change per day? Are the infant's bowel movements comfortable? Is the urine stream forceful and straight?

◆ Sleep patterns

How is the baby sleeping? Is the baby sleeping in a prone position? What has been the longest time the baby has slept during the night? How well are you sleeping? Do you hold or rock the baby to sleep or do you put the baby into the crib while awake? Determine the total number of hours of sleep, day and night cycles, the frequency of nighttime awakenings, and the impact of these cycles on other household members.

◆ Behavior and development

How would you describe your baby? What do you enjoy about your infant? What characteristics of your baby are difficult for you?

Determine the amount of crying, diurnal patterns, responses of the parents and other caregivers, and the impact that the crying is having on the household.

What are some of the new things your baby can do (see Box, Typical Developmental Progress at 2 Months)?

How does the infant relate to the mother, father, siblings, other caregivers, and relatives?

Questions about the family

◆ Family relationships

Have there been any changes in the family or household constellation?

Have there been any recent stresses, illnesses, or crises since the last visit?

What are the work schedules of the parents?

Many mothers who work outside the home return to their jobs at 6 to 12 weeks postpartum. Discuss the number of hours and schedule that parents work and their attitudes, beliefs, and struggles related to work.

Typical Developmental Progress at 2 Months

- *motor skills:* holds head temporarily erect; briefly holds a rattle
- *sensory skills:* tracks and follows objects visually; looks at faces in line of vision; responds to sounds by becoming quiet and alert
- *communication skills:* coos (makes musical, vowel-like sounds); parents may notice differentiated crying for differing needs
- *social skills:* smiles socially; begins to respond to voice by cooing; may begin to relate differentially to mother, father, siblings, other caregivers

What child care arrangements have been made?

How do the siblings relate to the infant?

Do the parents think they have enough private time?

Are there any special concerns about other family members (particularly about abuse of alcohol or other drugs or use of excessive punishment or violence)?

How is the mother doing? Does she have enough energy to resume her usual activities and responsibilities?

Physical Examination With Behavioral Observations

Measurements: *measure and plot percentiles*

- ◆ Height
- ◆ Weight
- ◆ Head circumference

General physical examination

To keep the infant as comfortable as possible, perform the less invasive procedures first. Observe, then palpate the infant. A stethoscope should be used before an otoscope or tongue depressor.

As part of the complete physical examination, carefully observe the infant for anatomic anomalies and evidence of the presence of congenital malformations. Look for flat areas on the occiput. Check the red reflex. Carefully examine the musculoskeletal system including the following: hips for subluxation, dislocation, limited abduction, or asymmetrical buttocks creases;

torticollis; and metatarsus adductus. A cardiac murmur may be detected initially at this age.

Continue to observe the interactions between the caregivers and the infant.

Assess hearing.

Observe developmental progress

Observe the infant for milestones if they are not well documented by history. Observe the infant's temperament, especially the abilities to cuddle and interact socially (see supplement on Individual Differences, p 223). Model social interactions for the parents if there are concerns about their responsiveness to the infant.

Note significant variations in the infant's development that warrant referral for full developmental assessment and/or early intervention, such as not smiling, not lifting the head, not responding to sound, or having abnormal muscle tone.

Screening Procedures

If the infant was premature or had a low birth weight, significant hemolysis, or excessive blood loss, a hematocrit or hemoglobin value may be indicated at this visit.

Formulation and Plan

Strengths of the Family and Infant

Speak positively and honestly about the physical, developmental, and temperamental strengths of the baby. "Look at how responsive the baby is to your voice."

Health Maintenance

Immunizations

Inform parents about the benefits and risks of immunizations that are administered at this visit. Parents should read the Vaccine Information Statements.* Answer any questions the parents may have. Ask whether the infant had any reactions to previous hepatitis B immunizations; record information in detail. Immunizations should include the following: the first dose of diphtheria, tetanus,

---

*Vaccine Information Statements can be obtained from the AAP.

and pertussis (DTaP or DTP; DTaP is preferred) vaccine, the first dose of inactivated poliovirus vaccine (IPV; the use of oral poliovirus vaccine [OPV] is not recommended except in special circumstances), the first dose of *Haemophilus influenzae* type b conjugate vaccine, and the second dose of hepatitis B vaccine (or the first dose if not given earlier). Remind parents that immunosuppressed persons should not be in direct contact with an infant after immunization with OPV. The first dose of pneumococcal conjugate vaccine should be given at this visit.

See the current Recommended Childhood Immunization Schedule.

Fever and irritability are common sequelae for DTP but less common for DTaP immunizations. Giving the infant one dose (10 to 15 mg/kg per dose) of acetaminophen in the office or on arrival home and a second dose 4 hours later reduces their incidence and severity. Warm compresses can be placed at the injection sites. If fever and irritability continue, acetaminophen may be given every 4 hours. Inform the parents to consult a physician if significant fever or irritability lasts longer than 24 hours.

Anticipatory guidance

◆ Nutrition

Encourage breastfeeding provided the infant and mother are doing well. Discuss the option of pumping or manually expressing milk if the mother has returned to work outside the home and the infant is not available to her. The infant should be fed about every 3 to 4 hours during the day and at longer intervals at night.

Mothers who breastfeed often comment about periods of high demand from their infants, which may indicate a growth spurt; the number of feedings may gradually diminish to four per day. Mothers who plan to return to work may introduce a daily bottle of expressed milk or formula at this age.

Vitamin D supplementation (400 IU/d) should be considered for exclusively breastfed children with dark pigmented skin or those who are not exposed to sunlight, particularly in northern states and countries during the winter months. Fluoride supplementation depends on the infant's water intake and on fluoride levels in the water supply.

Suggest iron supplementation for premature or anemic infants. The dose of supplemental elemental iron should not exceed 2 mg/kg/d for preterm infants, up to a maximum of 15 mg/d. Only a 1-month supply of the supplement should be in the house to reduce the risk of accidental poisoning.

The infant should not be fed honey or corn syrup until 12 months of age because of their association with infant botulism.

There is no nutritional advantage to feeding the infant solid foods before 4 to 6 months of age, when digestive processes and oropharyngeal motor skills have matured, and when foods are less likely to cause allergic reactions.

◆ Elimination

It is normal for an infant to have four to six wet diapers per day; the number of stools per day depends on the type of feeding — typically at least one stool per day for bottle-fed babies and greater variability for breastfed babies. Some babies may have one stool every 2 or 3 days without discomfort. Daily bowel movements are not necessary.

◆ Sleep patterns

Sleeping patterns of infants vary significantly. Sixteen hours or more of sleep per day is normal for infants.

Encourage establishing a diurnal rhythm of sleep and feeding. Encourage parents to put infants into the crib while still awake.

◆ Development and behavior

In the next 2 months expect increased smiling, vocalization, head control, and reaching (see Box, Typical Developmental Progress at 4 Months, p 43). The responsiveness of the infant to stimuli is important. Of concern are infants who appear apathetic or respond poorly to stimuli.

◆ Social/family relationships

Reinforce the parents' desire to play with, talk to, and cuddle their infant. Infants of this age are generally content with all caring adults.

Parents should explore the needs and behavior of other siblings. It is important that each parent spend time, even a few minutes, individually with each child daily.

Advise parents whose children need child care to obtain references for nonfamily caregivers or child care centers.

Parents individually or as a couple may need some time free from the responsibility of child care, particularly if the child is particularly challenging.

Maternal postpartum depression may have a detrimental effect on the behavior and development of the infant. Any indications of depression such as sad mood, feelings of hopelessness and helplessness, or vegetative signs should be explored fully and a mental health referral considered.

Encourage parents to preserve individual and family social activities and to get extra help and support from friends or members of their extended family. Parenting an infant is a demanding job!

◆ **Injury prevention**

Reinforce with parents the importance of car safety restraints. When the infant seat is being used as a carrier outside the car, place it on the ground or floor to prevent the infant from falling.

The infant should be carefully supervised during any contact with pets.

Infants should not be left unattended on a bed or table because they begin rolling over typically at 3 to 4 months of age.

Infants should not be held while a parent is drinking a hot liquid or smoking because they begin reaching and grabbing at 3 to 4 months of age.

Infant toys should be too big to swallow, unbreakable, and free of small detachable parts or sharp edges because infants take the objects they grab to their mouths.

Parents should be urged to maintain a smoke-free home and car. Environmental tobacco smoke is a serious health hazard, especially to infants and young children with respiratory problems such as asthma, recurrent ear infections, or bronchopulmonary dysplasia.

Guns in the home are a danger to the family. If a gun is kept in the home, advise parents to store the gun and ammunition in locked, separate locations. (Pediatricians and other child health care professionals are urged to inform parents about the dangers of guns in and outside the home. The AAP recommends that pediatricians incorporate questions about guns into their patient history taking and urge parents who possess guns to remove them, especially handguns, from the home.) Discuss other strategies for violence prevention.

Playpens may create an island of safety for an infant 3 months of age or older, particularly those in busy environments. Children should not spend excessive amounts of time in the playpen or swing.

Sunscreen is essential if the infant will be exposed to direct sunlight.

Teach parents the appropriate use of the emergency medical system (see Appendix E, Preparing Parents for Emergency Medical Services: A Parents' Guide). Inform parents of the importance of providing consent for emergency treatment when they are unavailable.

Suggest that parents learn CPR for infants and children.

Reinforce proper infant sleep positioning and environment.

Reinforce the need for smoke detectors in the home.

Problems and Plans

Review all issues and plans for addressing them (eg, recurrent coughing and urging parents to stop smoking).

Closing the Visit

◆ Have your goals been met for this visit? Are there any issues of concern we missed? New concerns raised late in the visit may require an additional scheduled visit before the next routine health maintenance visit.

◆ Set a time for the next appointment. Remind parents that during the next visit immunizations will be given.

◆ Indicate how to contact the office should any concerns arise prior to the next scheduled visit.

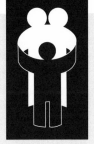

Health Supervision: 4-Month-Old Visit

Health Assessment

By 4 months babies are usually sleeping less, crying less, and smiling more than they had been. They are delighted with their parents, brothers and sisters, and other adults when they talk to them, and they reward this attention with smiles, squeals, and laughs. At this age babies are becoming more curious about their environment and look around eagerly at anything new or stimulating.

Interview With Behavioral Observations

Throughout the interview and physical examination, observe the parents' attitude toward the infant and the relationship among the caregivers and the baby.

Welcoming questions

How is your family? How is the baby? What particular issues or concerns do you want to discuss at this visit?

Check on the status of issues discussed at the previous visit.

Specific questions about the infant

◆ **Nutrition**

How is breastfeeding going? How often and how long does the baby feed? Are you giving the infant supplements of formula, vitamins, or fluoride? If the parents are bottle-feeding their infant, how many ounces does the baby drink in 24 hours? What are your plans about feeding the baby solid foods?

♦ **Elimination**

How many wet and dirty diapers does the infant have per day? Is the infant having any problems urinating or having bowel movements? What is the quality of the infant's urine stream?

♦ **Sleep patterns**

How is the baby sleeping? How many hours per day? How are you sleeping?

Determine the total number of hours the infant sleeps, day and night cycles, the number of nighttime awakenings, and the impact these cycles have on other household members.

♦ **Behavior and development**

How would you describe your baby? What do you enjoy about your infant? What characteristics of your baby are difficult for you? What are some of the new things your baby can do (see Box, Typical Developmental Progress at 4 Months)?

♦ **Social/family issues**

Does the mother rest when the baby naps? How does the infant relate to others — mother, father, siblings, alternative caregivers, relatives?

Questions about the family

♦ **Family relationships**

Have there been any changes in the family or household constellation? Have there been recent stresses, illnesses, or crises since last visit? What are the work schedules of the parents? What child care arrangements have been made?

What is your level of comfort and confidence with the child care arrangements? How do the siblings relate to the infant? Do the parents feel they have enough private time? Are there any special concerns about other family members, particularly abuse of alcohol or other drugs or use of excessive punishment or violence? How is the mother doing since the birth of the child? What is her energy level? Has she been able to resume her usual activities and responsibilities?

Typical Developmental Progress at 4 Months

- *motor skills:* holds head erect, raises body using arms from prone position, may roll prone to supine and supine to prone, may support weight on legs

- *fine motor skills:* reaches for and grabs objects, puts hands together, plays with hands, grabs a rattle, releases objects voluntarily

- *sensory skills:* tracks and follows objects visually to 180°, responds to sounds at least by becoming quiet and alert

- *communication skills:* coos reciprocally, expresses needs through differentiated crying, blows bubbles, may make "raspberry" sounds

- *social skills:* smiles readily in social settings, may laugh or squeal, differentiates individuals (mother, father, siblings, strangers)

Physical Examination With Behavioral Observations

Measurements: *measure and plot percentiles*

- ◆ Height

- ◆ Weight

- ◆ Head circumference

Discuss growth in length and weight with parents; demonstrate growth by showing parents the growth chart.

General physical examination

To keep the infant as comfortable as possible, perform the less invasive procedures first. Observe, then palpate the infant. A stethoscope should be used before an otoscope or tongue depressor.

As part of a complete physical examination, carefully observe the infant for congenital malformations. Check the infant's red reflex. Carefully examine the musculoskeletal system including the following: hips for subluxation, dislocation, limited abduction, or asymmetrical buttocks creases; torticollis; and metatarsus adductus. Listen carefully for a heart murmur. Assess hearing.

Observations of behavior and development

Continue to observe the quality of interactions among the caregivers and infant.

Observe the infant for appropriate milestones if they are not well documented by history (see Box, Typical Developmental Progress at 4 Months).

Observe the infant's temperament, especially the infant's abilities to cuddle, be calmed, and interact socially (see supplement on Individual Differences, p 223).

Model social interactions for the parents, especially if there are concerns about their responsiveness to the infant.

Screening Procedures

If the infant was premature or had a low birth weight, significant hemolysis, or excessive blood loss, a hematocrit or hemoglobin value may be obtained at this visit.

Formulation and Plan

Strengths of the Family and Infant

Speak positively and honestly about the physical, developmental, and temperamental strengths of the baby. "She seems like a happy and responsive little girl."

Health Maintenance

Immunizations

Inform parents about the benefits and risks of the immunizations to be administered at this visit. Parents should read the Vaccine Information Statements.* Answer any questions the parents may have. Ask whether the infant had any reactions to the previous immunizations; record information in detail. During this visit, administer the second doses of diphtheria, tetanus, and pertussis vaccine (DTaP or DTP; DTaP is preferred), inactivated poliovirus (IPV) vaccine (the use of oral poliovirus vaccine [OPV] is not recommended except in special circumstances), *Haemophilus influenzae* type b conjugate vaccine. Remind parents that immunosuppressed persons should not be in direct contact with the infant after immunization with OPV. The second dose of hepatitis B vaccine may be

*Vaccine Information Statements can be obtained from the AAP.

given if it was not administered earlier. The second dose of pneumococcal conjugate vaccine should be given at this visit.

See the current Recommended Childhood Immunization Schedule.

Use of antibiotics

Discuss upper respiratory tract infections (URIs) and judicious antibiotic use. Inform parents that (1) an average of six URIs per year is expected; (2) some infants will require antibiotic therapy, most will not; (3) colds are caused by viral infections; they will not respond to an antibiotic, but will get better without therapy; (4) unnecessary antibiotic use may increase the risk that their child will carry or become infected with resistant strains of bacteria; (5) for each URI, the possible benefits of antibiotics must be weighed against this risk; (6) children with URIs who are well enough to participate in activities can attend day care — antibiotics do not influence the transmissibility of colds.

Anticipatory guidance

◆ Nutrition

The number of feedings generally has been reduced to four or five per day. Bottle-fed infants can take up to 32 oz per day. Periods of high demand may indicate a growth spurt.

Vitamin D supplementation (400 IU/d) should be continued for exclusively breastfed children with dark pigmented skin or those who are not exposed to sunlight, particularly during the winter months. Fluoride supplementation depends on fluoride levels in the water supply and the infant's water intake.

The introduction of solid foods can begin at 4 to 6 months of age. Bottle-fed infants should continue receiving formula with iron. Breastfed infants should receive supplemental iron or iron-containing foods by 6 months of age. Advise parents to introduce new foods one at a time at 3- to 4-day intervals, starting with iron-fortified rice cereal.

Infants should not be fed honey or corn syrup until 12 months of age because of its association with infant botulism.

◆ Elimination

Stooling patterns may change with the introduction of solid foods. Stooling should be comfortable for the baby.

◆ Sleep patterns

Sleeping tends to become more regular after the child reaches 3 months of age. Many infants sleep through the night and take three naps. Parents of those who do not may be tired and frustrated.

Up to 16 hours of sleep per day is normal.

Encourage parents to establish a diurnal rhythm of sleeping and feeding.

◆ Developmental progress

Infants of this age are generally content with all caring adults. Colic typically resolves by 3 months of age. Persistent colic may warrant evaluation of the child, family, or environment.

In the next 2 months expect increased amounts of laughing, vocalization, reaching, and grabbing. Infants often begin sitting unassisted at about 6 months of age.

The responsiveness of the infant to stimuli is important. Of concern are infants who are apathetic or respond poorly to stimuli. The unpredictability of infants at this age may also be difficult for parents.

◆ Social/family relationships

Reinforce the parents' desire to play with, talk to, and cuddle the infant. Both parents should develop a unique relationship with the infant.

Parents should explore the needs and behavior of other siblings and spend time, even a few minutes, individually with each child daily. Explore how much time parents spend away from their infant and their feelings about separation.

Many mothers who work outside of the home have returned to their jobs. In addition to the number of hours and the schedule that the parents work, discuss their attitudes, beliefs, and stresses related to work.

Suggest that parents make unannounced visits to their child's caregivers to evaluate the care provided.

Sibling rivalry often becomes more apparent after the infant has been in the home for a while.

Parents individually or as a couple may need some time free from the responsibility of child care, particularly if the child is very challenging.

Maternal postpartum depression lasting more than 2 months may have a detrimental effect on the behavior and development of the infant. Any indications of maternal depression such as sad mood, feelings of hopelessness and helplessness, or significant fatigue should be explored fully, and referral to a mental health professional considered.

◆ **Injury prevention**

Reinforce with parents the importance of car safety restraints. When the infant seat is being used as a carrier outside the car, place it on the ground or floor to prevent the infant from falling.

Infants this age can roll front to back and back to front and therefore should not be left unattended on a bed or table.

Because infants reach and grab, they should not be held while a parent is drinking a hot liquid or smoking. Sharp and breakable items should be out of reach.

Infant toys should be too big to swallow, unbreakable, and free of small detachable parts or sharp edges because infants take the objects they grab to their mouths.

Parents should be urged to maintain a smoke-free home and car. Environmental tobacco smoke is a serious health hazard, especially to infants and young children with respiratory problems such as asthma, recurrent ear infections, or bronchopulmonary dysplasia.

Guns in the home are a danger to the family. If a gun is kept in the home, advise parents to store the gun and ammunition in locked, separate locations. (Pediatricians and other child health care professionals are urged to inform parents about the dangers of guns in and outside the home. The AAP recommends that pediatricians incorporate questions about guns into their patient history taking and urge parents who possess guns to remove them, especially handguns, from the home.) Discuss other strategies for violence prevention.

Playpens may create an island of safety for the infant, particularly in busy environments, and should also encourage exploration. Children should not spend excessive amounts of time in a playpen or swing.

The infant should not be exposed to direct sunlight without sunscreen.

Advise parents that infant exercise programs and swim classes are not necessary.

The infant's contact with pets should be supervised carefully.

Reinforce proper infant sleep positioning and environment.

Reinforce the need for smoke detectors in the home.

Problems and Plans

Review other issues and plans to address each of them (eg, frequent nighttime wakening and learning to fall asleep in the crib instead of being held).

Closing the Visit

◆ Have your goals been met for this visit? Are there any issues of concern we missed? New concerns raised late in the visit may require an additional scheduled visit before the next routine health maintenance visit.

◆ Set a time for the next appointment.

◆ Indicate how to contact the office should any concerns arise prior to the next scheduled visit.

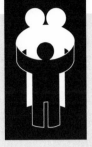

Health Supervision: 6-Month-Old Visit

Health Assessment

Six months is often called the Golden Age of infancy. Babies this age are still easy to keep in one place since they don't usually yet crawl. They are generally happy, love to interact with people, smile, and laugh easily. These babies show clearly how specially attached they are to their parents, sometimes even resisting being with baby-sitters or grandparents.

Interview With Behavioral Observations

Throughout the interview observe the parents' interactions with the baby and the relationship between the parents.

Welcoming questions

How is the baby? How are you? What particular issues do you want to discuss at this visit?

Check on the status of issues addressed at the last visit.

Specific questions about the infant

♦ **Nutrition**
How are feedings going? How often and how much milk does the baby take? Have you started any solid foods? Which ones? How often? Any problems? Is the baby still getting fluoride? Vitamins?

49

◆ **Elimination**
Any problems with urination or bowel movements?

◆ **Sleep patterns**
How much is the baby sleeping now? Does the baby go to sleep easily (both for naps and in the evening) and sleep through the night?

◆ **Behavior and development**
What is a typical day like with the baby? What are some new things the baby can do (see Box, Typical Developmental Progress at 6 Months). What does the family enjoy most about the baby? How would you describe the baby's personality?

Questions about the family

◆ **Family relationships**
How is the family doing? Have there been any recent stresses, illnesses, or crises since the last visit? How is each member of the family getting along with the baby? What are the work schedules of each parent? What are the child care arrangements? Do they seem satisfactory? How is the child care divided up among parents or others at home? Do the parents occasionally go out, leaving the infant with a baby-sitter? Is there any concern about alcohol or other drug abuse or violence in the family?

Physical Examination With Behavioral Observations

Continue to observe the interaction between the parents and the infant; does the infant show pleasure with the parents? Do the parents anticipate the baby's needs?

Typical Developmental Progress at 6 Months

◆ *motor skills:* holds head high when prone, raises body up on his or her hands, holds head steady when pulled up to sit, rolls over, sits with support

◆ *fine motor skills:* plays with his or her hands, holds a rattle, tries to obtain small objects with a raking movement, transfers objects from one hand to another

◆ *communication skills:* follows parents and objects visually to 180°, turns head toward sounds and familiar voices, babbles, laughs, squeals, takes initiative in vocalizing and babbling at others, imitates sounds, plays by making sounds

◆ *social skills:* initiates social contact by smiling, cooing, laughing, squealing; looks at, recognizes, and studies parents and other caregivers; shows pleasure and excitement with interactions with parents and other caregivers; may be displeased when a parent moves away or a toy is removed

Measurements: *measure and plot percentiles*

- ◆ Height
- ◆ Weight
- ◆ Head circumference

General physical examination

To keep the infant as comfortable as possible, perform the least invasive procedures first. Observe, then palpate the infant. The stethoscope should be used before the otoscope.

As part of the complete physical examination, check the infant's vision. Does the infant respond visually to movement? Check for conjugate gaze and symmetrical light reflex. Does the infant respond to sounds? Listen carefully for a heart murmur. Examine the infant for an abdominal mass and hip dislocation.

Observe developmental status

Observe the infant for age-appropriate achievements — especially for those not mentioned by the parents. Speak positively about the baby's behavior and developmental skills. "Very responsive ... good muscle strength and tone." The infant should be sitting alone (with or without support), reaching for toys, vocalizing, and socially responsive.

Screening Procedures

A sickle cell preparation should be done if indicated.

Formulation and Plan

Strengths of the Family and Infant

Speak positively and honestly about the baby's temperament development and physical findings. "Good weight gain! .... Good tone!" "Look how responsive he is!" Acknowledge the parents' strengths. If siblings are present compliment them as you observe their developmental skills in the office.

Health Maintenance

Immunizations

Ask about any reactions to previous immunizations; record information in detail. Parents should have read the Vaccine Information Statements*; review the benefits and risks of the immunizations and answer any questions the parent may have. The infant should receive the third dose of diphtheria, tetanus, and pertussis vaccine (DTaP or DTP; DTaP is preferred), inactivated poliovirus vaccine (IPV; the use of oral poliovirus vaccine [OPV] is not recommended except in special circumstances), Haemophilus influenzae type b vaccine, and hepatitis B vaccine (if due). Remind parents that immunosuppressed persons should not be in direct contact with an infant after immunization with OPV. The third dose of pneumococcal conjugate vaccine should be given at this visit.

See the current Recommended Childhood Immunization Schedule.

Giving the infant one dose of acetaminophen at the office or on arrival home and a second dose 4 hours later reduces the likelihood of fever and irritability.

Anticipatory guidance

◆ **Nutrition**

Breastfeeding may be continued. Infants should not be placed in cribs with bottles to reduce risks of nursing bottle caries and otitis media. Bottles should not be used as pacifiers.

Offer the infant sips of drinks from a cup.

The infant should start being fed solid foods. The infant may be fed two or three meals daily, with a new food introduced at 3- to 4-day intervals. Iron-fortified cereal should be included in the infant's diet.

Remind parents not to feed the infant honey or corn syrup until 12 months of age because of the risk of infant botulism.

Administer vitamin D (400 IU/d) for breastfed infants with dark pigmented skin or those not exposed to sunlight.

Continue fluoride and vitamin supplementation (if indicated).

◆ **Elimination**

Changing the diaper: If the parent is having difficulty, recommend the use of a toy or a musical mobile to occupy the infant. Allow the baby to explore his or her genitalia during diaper changing.

*Vaccine Information Statements can be obtained from the AAP.

◆ **Sleep patterns**
Most babies usually nap twice a day. Separation anxiety may cause the infant
to resist going to sleep. A special stuffed animal or blanket may be helpful.
Babies should be put to bed while still awake. If the baby wakes up during
the night, he or she should be comforted but not fed or played with (see
supplement on Sleep Problems, p 219).

◆ **Development and behavior**
As a result of increasing recognition of others in the environment and
the development of "object permanence," infants may resist staying with
anyone other than their parents, sometimes even the grandparents or
favorite baby-sitter. Parents should not trick the child or sneak away to
keep the infant from crying. Peek-a-boo is a favorite game at this stage
as it gives the child a chance to practice the comings and goings of parents
and other favorite people. Parents should reassure the child that they will
return.

Talk with parents about safe, inexpensive, age-appropriate toys to aid in the
child's development.

◆ **Language development**
Parents can stimulate language development by talking to and responding
to the baby's sounds and by reading aloud to the child.

◆ **Motor development**
During the second half of the baby's first year, the growth in independent
mobility is a primary achievement. The baby will be learning to get to a
sitting position and sit alone without support, to crawl, and perhaps to
pull up to a standing position before the next scheduled health supervision
visit. In the realm of fine motor dexterity the pincer grasp is mastered by
9 months of age, when the baby is able to bring the tips of his or her
thumb and index finger together to manipulate a small object.

◆ **Injury prevention**
Because the baby is becoming more active and is therefore more prone to
injury, remind parents that the baby needs constant attention. To "childproof" the home, remove small objects (pins, buttons, pennies) from the
floor; keep plastic wrappers, plastic bags, and balloons out of reach.

All medications (including acetaminophen, vitamins, iron preparations, and
birth control pills) and household poisons (furniture polish, detergents,
and drain cleaners) should be kept in locked cabinets.

Make sure the parents have the telephone number of the local poison
control center (or if one is not available, the emergency department or
physician's 24-hour telephone number); advise them to tape this number

to their telephone. Advise parents to have syrup of ipecac in their home, but they should never use this antidote without medical advice. Remind parents to review the instructions regarding poisonings with anyone who comes into the house to baby-sit and to supply the emergency telephone number to anyone who cares for the baby in another home.

Teach parents the appropriate use of the emergency medical system (see Appendix E, Preparing Parents for Emergency Medical Services: A Parents' Guide). Inform parents of the importance of providing consent for emergency treatment when they are unavailable.

The infant should be protected from hot liquids and surfaces. Appliances such as irons and curling irons should not be within the baby's reach.

Warn parents that the baby may pull down the tablecloths, lamps, drawers, and dangling electrical cords while attempting to stand.

The infant should never be left unattended on the bed or changing table, in a tub of water, or at the water's edge.

Plastic plugs should be inserted into electrical outlets. The junction points of extension cords should be insulated with electrical tape.

The baby's skin should be protected from the sun with hat and clothing and sunscreen approved for infants 6 months or older (UVB protection of at least SPF 15 plus UVA protection).

Car seats should be used on all trips.

The use of infant walkers should be avoided; if they are used, the infant must be watched carefully; a walker is not a playpen and should never be used in an area with stairs.

Guns in the home are a danger to the family. If a gun is kept in the home, advise parents to store the gun and ammunition in locked, separate locations. (Pediatricians and other child health care professionals are urged to inform parents about the dangers of guns in and outside the home. The AAP recommends that pediatricians incorporate questions about guns into their patient history taking and urge parents who possess guns to remove them, especially handguns, from the home.) Discuss other strategies for violence prevention.

Infant swim classes are not recommended. Parents may have a false sense of security if their child participates in infant swim classes; children are not developmentally ready for swim classes until after their fourth birthday. When an adult plays with an infant in water, the water temperature should be appropriate, the infant should not be submerged, and fecal contamination should be controlled. Each infant should be paired with a responsible adult within an arm's length (the adult should be able to touch the infant at all times). If the parents decide to enroll their child in swim classes, they should be advised that the instructor must be certified in CPR.

Reinforce proper infant sleep positioning and environment.

Reinforce the need for UV protection.

Reinforce the need for smoke detectors in the home.

Problems and Plans

Discuss all problems identified and plans to address each of them.

Closing the Visit

◆ **Have your goals for this visit been met? Are there other issues you want to discuss? Dealing with new concerns raised at this point may require scheduling a visit sooner than the next routine visit.**

◆ **Set a time for the next appointment.**

◆ **Indicate your availability should any concerns arise prior to the next scheduled visit.**

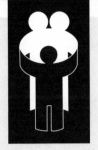

Health Supervision: 9-Month-Old Visit

Health Assessment

A big change occurs in babies between 6 and 9 months of age. Now they are usually able to get around on their own, they have developed an efficient way to pick up small objects and get them to their mouths, and they have begun to develop a mind of their own. The normal hesitancy of babies this age to let their parents out of sight may complicate and prolong some daily routines.

Interview With Behavioral Observations

Throughout the interview and physical examination, observe the parents' attitude toward the infant and the relationship between the caregivers and infants, both in verbal interchange and nonverbal behavior.

Welcoming questions

How is your baby? How are you? What particular issues or concerns do you want to discuss at this visit?

Check on the status of issues addressed at the previous visit.

Specific questions about the infant

◆ Nutrition

How is the infant's appetite? How often is the baby nursing? How much formula or juice does the baby drink? What finger foods is the infant eating? What other foods, and how much? Is the infant drinking from a cup?

◆ Elimination

Any problems urinating or having bowel movements?

◆ Sleep patterns

How is the infant sleeping? Does the infant take naps? What time does the infant go to bed? Does the infant wake up at night?

◆ Behavior and development

What is your infant like these days? Have there been changes in personality? Describe the infant's activity level. How does the child respond to "no" — by throwing a tantrum or breath holding? Is it easy to distract the child from unsafe or undesirable activities?

How does the child respond to separation? What are some of the new things your baby can do (see Box, Typical Developmental Progress at 9 Months)?

Ask how discipline was handled in the parents' families. What are the household rules the parents have agreed on? What will they do when the child breaks a rule or touches a forbidden object? Do the parents agree on how to discipline their child?

◆ Questions about family circumstances

Have there been any changes in the family or household constellation? Have there been any recent stresses, illnesses, or crises since the last visit? What are the work schedules of the parents? What are their attitudes and stresses related to working? What are the child care arrangements? Are the parents comfortable with their child care arrangements? How are the siblings getting along with the infant? Do the parents each feel they have enough private time? Are any changes in the family anticipated between now and the next visit in 3 months? If so, how will they be handled?

◆ Injury prevention

Do you have gates blocking off all staircases? Where are the smoke alarms installed? When did you last check their functioning? Is your water heater thermostat set at 120°F? Are there guns in the home? Where are they stored? How do you keep medications away from the child? Where do you keep household cleaning products? Are there any special concerns about other family members, particularly concerning alcohol or other drug abuse or excessive punishment or violence?

Typical Developmental Progress at 9 Months

- *gross motor skills:* sits well, crawls, creeps on hands, may walk holding onto the furniture
- *fine motor skills:* picks up small objects using a thumb and index finger, brings hands to mouth, feeds self, bangs objects together
- *cognitive skills:* becomes interested in the trajectory of falling objects, searches for hidden objects
- *communication skills:* responds to own name, participates in verbal requests such as "wave bye-bye" or "where is mama or dada?" understands a few words such as "no" or "bye-bye"; imitates vocalizations, babbles using several syllables
- *social skills:* enjoys social games with familiar adults such as peek-a-boo and patty-cake, may react to unfamiliar adults with anxiety or fear

Physical Examination With Behavioral Observations

Infants at 9 months of age are at the height of stranger awareness. The intensity of the infants' responses to strangers is highly variable. Although they may have been friendly and cooperative at the previous visit they are far more likely to become upset with the physical examination at this age. The clinician can minimize this reaction by approaching the infant very slowly, by examining the infant in a parent's arms, by first touching the infant's shoe or leg and gradually moving to the chest, and by distracting the infant with a toy or stethoscope during examination.

Measurements: *measure and plot percentiles*

- ◆ Height
- ◆ Weight
- ◆ Head circumference

General physical examination

To keep the infant as comfortable as possible, perform the less invasive procedures first. Observe, then palpate the infant. A stethoscope should be used before an otoscope or tongue depressor.

As part of the complete physical examination, check the infant's eyes for strabismus and red reflex. Check the pattern and degree of tooth eruption. Assess the range of movement at the hips, examining the infant for limited abduction. Check the descent of the testes. Neurological examination includes the downward parachute reaction, bilateral pincer grasp, and assessment of muscle tone. Assess hearing.

Observations of behavior and development

Continue to observe the interactions among the caregivers and the infant.

At this age, many infants begin to interact in a purposeful manner, play with toys, and cry when familiar caregivers leave the room.

Observe the infant for milestones that were not well documented by history. Observe the infant's sociability and attentiveness.

Note significant delays in development that warrant referral for a full developmental assessment and/or early intervention, such as poor muscle tone, absence of babbling, or little evidence of social interaction or communication.

Screening Procedures

A hemoglobin or hematocrit determination should be done at the 9-month or 12-month visit (preferably at the 9-month visit).

The risk for lead poisoning should be assessed using the assessment questions (see Box, Lead Toxicity Screening).

If the infant is at high risk for lead poisoning, a blood lead level should be measured at this visit.

For infants at high risk for tuberculosis, a tuberculin test using purified protein derivative (Mantoux) should be performed now or at the 12-month visit (see Appendix F, Recommendations for Tuberculosis Testing). It should be read in 48 to 72 hours.

Formulation and Plan

Strengths of the Family and Infant

Speak positively and honestly about the physical, developmental, and temperament strengths of the infant. "Look at how well your child is getting around."

Health Maintenance

Immunizations

Find out whether the infant had any reactions to the previous immunizations; record information in detail. No immunizations are due at this visit for infants whose vaccinations have been given on schedule. Check to ensure that the child's immunizations are up-to-date.

Lead Toxicity Screening

Questions to assess risk status for lead poisoning.

Does your child:

- spend time in buildings built before 1950 with peeling or chipping paint, including day care centers, preschools, or the homes of baby-sitters or relatives?

- live in or regularly visit buildings built before 1950 with recent, ongoing, or planned renovation or remodeling?

- have a brother or sister, housemate, or playmate being followed up or treated for lead poisoning (blood lead level >15 µg/dL)?

- frequently come in contact with an adult whose job or hobby involves exposure to lead, such as construction, welding, pottery, or other trades?

- live near an active lead smelter, battery recycling plant, or other industry likely to release lead?

If the answer to any of these questions is YES, the child is considered to be at risk of excessive lead exposure and should be screened with a blood lead test.

For more detailed management, see Appendix G and the AAP policy statement "Screening for Elevated Blood Lead Levels."

Anticipatory guidance

◆ Nutrition

Breastfeeding or formula should be continued, and the infant should be offered a variety of other foods and drinks. Most children need three or four feedings per day. Provide regular meal times and offer table foods, such as potatoes, soft carrots and peas, noodles, and fruits, as well as puréed foods of all kinds. Because most babies this age have mastered the "pincer grasp," they can pick up small objects successfully. This makes feeding themselves an enjoyable challenge!

Meals provide opportunities for social interaction as well as for nutrition. Infants can generally feed themselves toast, bread, and teething biscuits and can be encouraged to drink from a cup. Infants should be weaned from the bottle by 12 or 15 months.

◆ Elimination

Increasing diversity of foods leads to variation in stooling patterns. In many cases, constipation can be relieved by dietary changes (such as increases in eating certain fruits and vegetables, ie, apples and bananas tend to have binding effects, whereas prunes, plums, and apricots tend to have laxative effects). Toilet training should be delayed until about 2 years of age or later when the child is ready.

◆ Sleep patterns

Most infants take 2 daytime naps and sleep through the night by this age. Some infants who previously slept through the night may begin waking up during the night.

A regular bedtime routine should be established. The introduction of a familiar or favorite toy may help some infants fall back asleep. The infant should not be fed or played with if he or she awakens during the night. Brief periods of crying will encourage infants to settle themselves and resume sleep (see supplement on Sleep Problems, p 219).

◆ Behavioral developments

Increasing mobility and overall competence often lead to new challenges. This may be the first age at which parents consider the need for explicit disciplinary rules. Discuss discipline for the child (see supplement on Effective Discipline, p 225).

Distraction and diversion are typically successful disciplinary measures at this age. It is easier to change the environment than the child's behavior!

Discuss "separation anxiety." Many infants this age cry when parents leave their presence. Such behavior is normal and relates to their cognitive and social development. The behavior does not reflect that they are "spoiled." Infants grow socially and cognitively by separating from and reuniting with parents. For this reason, short or regular parent-child separations typically are helpful in teaching the infants that when parents go away they also come back.

If child care has not been used, this may be a difficult age to start.

Sibling rivalry may intensify at this age when the infant begins to crawl or walk and gain access to the toys and play space of his or her siblings. Parents can find themselves trapped between supporting the older child's need for privacy and protecting the infant from the older sibling's anger.

Parents should encourage infants to use their emerging language (vocalizing and imitating sounds) because the degree of vocal output is associated with the ability to learn language later. Some techniques to promote communication include imitating the infant's own sounds and playing social and interactive games. Parents should be encouraged to "narrate your life" as they interact with their infant. This is a good age to begin regular daily reading.

By this age, most parents need opportunities away from the responsibilities of parenting. Discuss to whom parents turn for support.

◆ **Injury prevention**

Review safety conditions in the home with parents. Parents should take the necessary precautions to prevent falls caused by the infant's increased mobility: use gates at stairwells, and install safety devices on windows and screens. Heavy and hot containers should be kept out of the reach of infants and children. As children pull themselves up onto furniture, they may grab and accidentally pull down tablecloths or other objects.

Sharp objects such as knives, scissors, tools, razor blades, and other hazardous items such as coins, glass objects, beads, pins, art objects, and medications should be kept in secure places.

The infant should be prevented from playing with electrical sockets or extension cords.

Infants should not be fed foods that may be easily aspirated such as peanuts, hot dogs, popcorn, frozen peas, candy corn, raw celery, or raw carrot sticks. Infants should be seated in a high chair and watched by an adult at all times while eating. The infant should not be allowed to play with a mouth full of food.

Make sure that the parents have the telephone number for the poison control center (or the pediatric emergency room or hot line telephone number). This number should be taped to the telephone and called to the attention of anyone who cares for the infant.

Syrup of ipecac should be on hand and stored in a safe place. Make sure all of the baby's caregivers are aware of the storage location. Advise parents to use this emesis-inducing drug only as directed by the poison control center or the physician.

Advise parents that toxic substances (eg, cleaning fluids, drain cleaners, paint thinner) should not be stored in empty soda bottles, glasses, or jars and should be kept in a locked cabinet out of reach of the child.

Guns in the home are a danger to the family. If a gun is kept in the home, advise parents to store the gun and ammunition in locked, separate locations. (Pediatricians and other child health care professionals are urged to inform parents about the dangers of guns in and outside the home. The AAP recommends that pediatricians incorporate questions about guns into their patient history taking and urge parents who possess guns to remove them, especially handguns, from the home.) Discuss other strategies for violence prevention.

The infant's car seat should be upgraded to a toddler car restraint when the infant weighs 20 lb.

Strongly advise parents against the use of infant walkers because of the danger of falls.

Reinforce the need for UV protection.

Reinforce the need for smoke detectors in the home.

Problems and Plans

Discuss problems that emerged during the visit and plans to address each of them. This is the time for written and verbal advice — as well as planning an evaluation for specific problems.

Closing the Visit

◆ **Have your goals been met for this visit?**

◆ **Are there any issues we missed? New concerns raised late in the visit may require an additional scheduled visit before the next routine health supervision visit. Prioritize the importance of a new concern.**

◆ **Set a time for the next appointment.**

◆ **Indicate how to contact the office should any concerns arise prior to the next scheduled visit.**

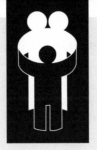

Health Supervision: 12-Month-Old Visit

Health Assessment

One-year-olds are entering toddlerhood. They are generally sure of themselves and attached to their parents and other important caregivers. They begin to venture out on their own, using their new mobility skills to explore the world beyond their crib or high chair. They have learned several ways to communicate through sounds and gestures, and they will expand these abilities dramatically over the next year.

Interview With Behavioral Observations

Throughout the interview and physical examination, observe the interactions of the parents and infant, noting both verbal interchanges and nonverbal behavior.

Welcoming questions

How is your infant? How are you? How is the rest of the family?

What particular issues do you want to discuss at this visit?

Check on the status of issues discussed at the previous visit.

Specific questions about the infant

◆ Nutrition

How is the infant's appetite? If the mother is nursing, how frequently? If the infant is being fed formula, how much? When do you plan to introduce cow's milk? How much and what kinds of puréed food is the infant eating? Is the infant eating finger foods? What ones, and how much? Is the infant drinking from a cup?

◆ Elimination

Is the infant having any problems urinating or having bowel movements?

◆ Sleep patterns

Does the infant go to bed at a regular time? What is the infant's bedtime routine? Does the infant wake up during the night? How much does the infant nap during the day?

◆ Behavior and development

What are some of the things your infant can do (see Box, Typical Developmental Progress at 12 Months)? What is your infant like these days? What things does your infant find fun to do? What are your infant's favorite toys? How does the infant respond to "no"? How does the infant respond to separations? What feedback have you had from the child care provider? Does the infant recognize parents and other regular caregivers?

What rules have you made in your home? Where is the infant allowed to go in the house? What is your infant allowed to touch or do? What happens if the infant "breaks" the rules? How were you punished when you were a child? How was your spouse or partner punished?

Questions about the family

◆ Family relationships and discipline

Who helps in caring for the baby? Have there been any changes in the family recently? Any new stresses? Any problems related to alcohol or other drug use or violence?

Who takes care of the baby during the day? What are the work situations and schedules of the parents?

How are the siblings getting along with the infant?

What private time has the primary caregiver been able to arrange since the baby's arrival?

Do the parents agree on how to discipline the child?

Are any changes in the family anticipated between now and the next visit in 3 months? If so, how will they be handled?

Typical Developmental Progress at 12 Months

- *motor skills:* sits without support, crawls, pulls self up and walks with support, feeds self using spoon or fingers, opposes thumb and index finger to grasp a small object ("pincer grasp")

- *cognitive skills:* plays with adult-like objects, eg, a comb, telephone, cooking equipment

- *communication skills:* plays peek-a-boo, patty-cake, waves good-bye, likes to look at pictures in books and magazines, points to animals or named body parts, imitates words, follows simple commands, eg, waves bye-bye or points when asked, "Where is mommy?"

◆ Injury prevention

Do you have gates blocking off all staircases? Where are the smoke alarms installed? When did you last check their functioning? Is your water heater thermostat set at 120°F? Are there guns in the home? Where are they stored? How do you keep medications away from the child? Where do you keep household cleaning products?

Physical Examination With Behavioral Observations

Continue to observe the interactions between the parents and child. Notice the reaction of the parents to the infant's expressions of fear or distress, smiling, vocalizations, and motor activity.

Measurements: *measure and plot percentiles*

- ◆ Height

- ◆ Weight

- ◆ Head circumference

General physical examination

Children at this age are uncomfortable about being restrained in their activity. The physical examination may be more successfully performed while the child is on a parent's lap or standing on the floor. Speaking directly to the child and taking a playful stance about the examination will make it easier for the child to cooperate. If the child becomes upset, it is helpful to remind the parent that this is an expected reaction at this age.

As part of the complete physical examination, perform the noninvasive proce-dures first, with the eyes, ears, nose, and mouth examined last. Check the infant for strabismus and red reflex. Note the pattern of tooth eruption. Check the descent of the testes. Check the range of motion of the hips, or the gait if the infant is walking. Check leg alignment and hip rotation for internal tibial torsion, external rotation contracture of the hip, and femoral anteversion. Assess hearing.

Observations of behavior and development

Observe the infant for developing landmarks that are not well-enough documented by history. Absent or diminished vocalization or mobility would be causes for further evaluation. Note the interactions and com-munication between the child and parent(s). Can the parent occupy and comfort the child? Is the child attentive and sociable?

Screening Procedures

A hemoglobin or hematocrit determination should be done at this visit if it was not done at the 9-month visit. If the infant is at high risk for lead poisoning, a lead level should be measured at this visit if it has not been done previously (see Appendix G, Lead Toxicity Screening). Federal Medicaid guidelines require children enrolled in the Medicaid program to have a lead level measurement at 1 and 2 years of age.

If high-risk factors for tuberculosis are present, a test using purified protein derivative (Mantoux) should be performed and read within 72 hours by a health professional (see Appendix F, Recommendations for Tuberculosis Testing).

Formulation and Plan

Strengths of the Family and Infant

Describe some of the child's new developmental achievements. Remind parents of the importance of their active modeling and positive interactions for the child's develop-ment, and compliment them on their concern and care for the infant.

Health Maintenance

Immunizations

Check to make sure that immunizations are up-to-date. The third dose of inacti-vated poliovirus vaccine may be administered at this visit if it was not given at the 6-month visit. (Oral poliovirus vaccine [OPV] is not recommended except under special circumstances; if use of OPV is necessary, remind parents that immunosuppressed persons should not be in direct contact with an infant after immunization with OPV.) The first dose of measles, mumps, rubella (MMR) may be given at this visit. Varicella immunization may be given at this visit. Make sure the parents have read the Vaccine Information Statements.* The fourth doses of *Haemophilus influenzae* type b and pneumococcal conjugate vaccines may be given at this visit. The third dose of hepatitis B vaccine should be given at this visit if it was not given at the 6-month visit.

See the current Recommended Childhood Immunization Schedule.

Use of antibiotics

Discuss upper respiratory tract infections (URIs) and judicious antibiotic use. Inform parents that (1) an average of six URIs per year is expected; (2) some infants will require antibiotic therapy, most will not; (3) colds are caused by viral infections; they will not respond to an antibiotic, but will get better without therapy; (4) unnecessary antibiotic use may increase the risk that their child will carry or become infected with resistant strains of bacteria; (5) for each URI, the possible benefits of antibiotics must be weighted against this risk; (6) children with URIs who are well enough to participate in activities can attend day care — antibiotics do not influence the transmissibility of colds.

Anticipatory guidance

◆ Nutrition

Many parents find that the appetites of infants diminish in the second year of life. Infants may also become pickier about what they like to eat. It is wise for parents to set clear routines and expectations about mealtimes and to avoid struggles about what and how much their children eat. Regular meals and scheduled snacks are preferable to snacking "on demand."

Babies are ready to be weaned from breastfeeding and bottle-feeding, and should be moving toward being fed entirely table foods. Formula can be discontinued. The fat, salt, and sugar content of the baby's food should be

---

*Vaccine Information Statements can be obtained from the AAP.

monitored and limited. Fluoride supplementation, if indicated, should continue. Nuts, hard candies, chewing gum, and hard raw fruits and vegetables should be avoided.

◆ Elimination

In most cases, toilet training should not be considered until the baby is at least 2 years old.

◆ Sleep patterns

The number of hours babies sleep varies. Infants should continue to have at least one nap during the day. It is important to establish a regular bedtime routine. If the infant is waking up in the middle of the night or having trouble settling down at bedtime, it is often helpful for parents to increase the structure of the bedtime routine and to clarify their expectation that the infant will stay in bed even if awake. Parents should be discouraged from allowing their children to join them in bed during the night unless cultural expectations or social circumstances support cosleeping. If cosleeping, mattress must be firm, no soft materials (pillows, comforters), and no smoking, alcohol, or drugs.

◆ Behavior and development

The child's temperament may seem very much the same as it did in infancy or may shift as the child gains increasing mastery over the environment. Parents should be attentive and appreciative of the child's drive toward increased autonomy. Some children start to "play favorites" between their parents; each parent should continue to have positive "one-on-one" interactions with the child, despite the child's current preferences. Appropriate toys for this age include blocks or rings, dolls, stuffed animals, and books with simple but realistic pictures.

◆ Social relationships

Despite the child's growing activity, cuddling and being held are still important contacts between the parents and child, as are talking and singing.

◆ Communication skills

Most children this age have a receptive vocabulary greater than their expressive vocabulary. They can follow simple commands and identify pictures in a book or body parts, although they may not yet be able to express themselves.

Most children this age can use "mama" and "dada" correctly. They may also have three to five additional recognizable words, as well as using unintelligible or meaningless "jargon" and other vocalizations.

Language skills develop quickly during the next 6 months. Parents can facilitate this remarkable development by speaking to the child in simple sentences and "labeling" commonly encountered items and actions with clear words and phrases. Labeling items in books and magazines is another way to encourage language development. Attempts by children to imitate these words should be celebrated and encouraged.

◆ **Cognitive skills**

Favorite toys include blocks that can be banged together and objects that can be stacked or put inside one another. Around this age children may begin to play imaginary or "pretend" games and to imitate parental activities such as sweeping or cooking.

◆ **Motor skills**

Around 1 year of age, infants begin to walk, then climb, then run. These achievements are inherently reinforcing for the child, and parents need to do little else than appreciate the immense accomplishment they represent. Fine motor development is less dramatic at this age and is most evident in the increasing ability of the infant to grasp and manipulate small objects and use a spoon. They may also increase the amount of finger foods they eat; and resist being fed puréed "baby food."

◆ **Discipline**

With newfound mobility and the drive for independence and autonomy, toddlers are eager to explore a wider radius. Parents should be encouraged to appreciate the need for rules and limits to be defined when there are threats to the infant's safety, property, or the orderliness of desired household routines.

Infants should come to expect that they will be noticed more for their appropriate behavior than for their undesirable behavior. Effective disciplinary actions, when necessary, include distraction, a stern restatement of the forbidden action (eg, "hitting is not allowed"), or a brief period of noninteraction ("time-out"). Suggestions for the management of temper tantrums are discussed in detail in the supplements (see Effective Discipline, p 225).

◆ **Family relationships**

It is important for parents to nurture their relationship in the interest of their children. If significant stresses are affecting the family, such as financial instability, marital conflict, unemployment, alcohol or other drug use, physical or emotional abuse, chronic illness or death of a family member, or lack of adequate social support, it may be appropriate to suggest that the family receive counseling or attend a peer support group.

◆ **Injury prevention**

Parents should be attentive to the dangers inherent in their infant's increased mobility. They should "childproof" their home and other places where the infant spends time, focusing on the following common threats:

Scalds from irons, liquids that have been heated and are sitting on top of the stove, and tap water that is too hot.

Ingestion of prescription or over-the-counter medications. All medications should be locked in a cabinet and out of the infant's reach. The poison control center's telephone number as well as syrup of ipecac should be conveniently located.

Ingestions of household cleaners, paint thinners, and drain cleaners. These items should also be inaccessible to the infant and stored in clearly marked containers that do not resemble food containers.

Ingestion of small toys or food items.

Falls from windows or down stairs. Windows and stairs should be guarded with railings or gates. The use of walkers should be discouraged.

Sunburn. Infants should be kept out of the sun at peak times (10:00 am to 3:00 pm) and should be protected with sunscreen at all times.

Drowning. Infants should be accompanied when in or near water at all times, even in a partially filled bathtub. A locked fence should surround a pool.

Motor vehicle injuries. Infants should continue to be restrained in an appropriate car seat at all times (car safety seats may face the front of the car beginning at 1 year of age and when the child weighs more than 20 lb); parents should also wear seat belts. Infants should not ride on tractors or lawn mowers or play near or in a driveway. Outdoor play areas should be enclosed or closely supervised.

Guns in the home. If a gun is kept in the home, advise parents to store the gun and ammunition in locked, separate locations. (Pediatricians and other child health care professionals are urged to inform parents about the dangers of guns in and outside the home. The AAP recommends that pediatricians incorporate questions about guns into their patient history taking and urge parents who possess guns to remove them, especially handguns, from the home.) Discuss other strategies for violence prevention.

Reinforce the need for UV protection.

Reinforce the need for smoke detectors in the home.

◆ **Other advice**
Parents should be taught the appropriate use of the medical emergency system (see Appendix E, Preparing Parents for Emergency Medical Services: A Parents' Guide). Inform parents of the importance of providing consent for emergency treatment when they are unavailable.

Parents should maintain a tobacco-free and drug-free environment.

Parents should not allow their infant in the bathroom unsupervised.

An infant's shoes should be flexible, inexpensive, and a good fit in both length and width. Shoes are needed only to protect the child's feet from sharp objects and the cold. Rigid shoes should be avoided. Shoes should not be altered with wedges and heels for treatment of flexible flat feet, toeing-in, or toeing-out. Many infants have toes that turn in at the age when they begin to walk.

Problems and Plans

Review other issues and plans to address each of them (eg, eating problems, skin problems such as eczema, helping the child with an impending divorce).

Closing the Visit

◆ **Have your goals for this visit been met?**

◆ **Are there any issues we missed? New concerns raised late in the visit may require an additional scheduled visit before the next routine health maintenance visit.**

◆ **Compliment the parents on how well the baby is doing and on how well they are parenting. Comment on a particular strength you see in the family.**

◆ **Set a time for the next appointment. If the MMR is not given at this visit, you may want to give the parents the MMR Vaccine Information Statements to read before the 15-month visit.**

◆ **Indicate how to contact the office should any concerns arise prior to the next scheduled visit.**

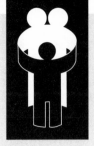

Health Supervision: 15-Month-Old Visit

Health Assessment

As toddlers become sure of their ability to move around their environment, they also find barriers to their continuing explorations. In order to keep them safe and to maintain order and balance in the family, the parents have to impose rules and limits on toddlers and frustrate some of their excitement. As toddlers acquire more independence physically, they also begin to assert their own will, resulting in their well-known temper tantrums and abundant challenges to their parents' patience and self-confidence.

Interview With Behavioral Observations

Observe the interactions between the parents and toddler throughout the interview. There may be opportunities to observe the parents' affection and their support for the toddler's new skills. The clinician and parent may communicate verbally with the toddler, teach the functional use of objects in play, and encourage autonomy.

Welcoming questions

How are you doing? How has your baby been? How is the family doing?

What are the particular issues you want to discuss at this visit?

Check on the status of issues addressed at the previous visit.

Specific questions about the baby

◆ Nutrition

Has your infant shown a decrease in appetite? Has your infant been eating anything that is not food (pica)?

◆ Elimination

Any problems with urination or bowel movements?

◆ Sleep patterns

Does your baby wake up during the night or experience difficulty going to sleep?

◆ Behavior and development

How would you describe your baby? What are some of the new things your baby is doing (see Box, Typical Developmental Progress at 15 Months)? How does your child show affection? Is your baby active, demanding, obstinate, or aggressive? How does he or she communicate?

Questions about the family

Is there a parent at home full-time? Who helps with child care? Have the parents observed the child care provider interacting with the baby? Is the arrangement well supervised and safe? Do the parents agree about how to raise their child? Have the parents discussed their child-rearing ideas and rules with other caregivers? How does the child's increasing independence make the parents feel?

Physical Examination With Behavioral Observations

Measurements: *measure and plot percentiles*

- ◆ Height
- ◆ Weight
- ◆ Head circumference

General physical examination

To keep the child as comfortable as possible, perform the less invasive procedures first. Much of the examination can be done in the parent's lap, preoccupying the toddler with a toy or examining instrument.

As part of the complete physical examination, observe the child's gait, check for hip dysplasia; examine the baby for hernias, strabismus, and abdominal masses. Check the baby's teeth. Assess vision and hearing.

Typical Developmental Progress at 15 Months

- *fine motor skills:* feeds self with fingers or a spoon, scribbles with crayons, stacks two blocks

- *cognitive skills:* shows functional understanding of objects (pretends to use a toy phone, holds a comb near hair)

- *communication skills:* says single words (approximately 5-15), uses unintelligible or meaningless words (jargon), communicates with gestures, points to one or two body parts on request, understands simple commands, points to designated pictures in books, listens to stories being read

- *social skills:* gives and takes toys, plays games with parents, communicates pleasure or displeasure, is interested in new experiences, tests parental limits or rules

Observations of behavior and development

Observe the child for milestones and temperament as previously discussed. Note that with increasing autonomy the infant may resist being examined. During the examination observe how the parents help or hinder the infant's ability to cope. Be concerned if the toddler is overly passive or uncommunicative, does not walk, has poor manual dexterity, does not talk, or appears to have poor comprehension.

Screening Procedures

A hemoglobin or hematocrit should be performed for children at risk. The risk for lead poisoning should be assessed using the assessment questions (see Appendix G, Lead Toxicity Screening). If the infant is at high risk, a blood lead level should be determined.

Check the child's immunization status and whether he or she had any reactions to previous immunizations or tuberculosis tests; record information in detail. If the child or community is at high risk for tuberculosis, a test using purified protein derivative (Mantoux) should be given if not previously done (see Appendix F, Recommendations for Tuberculosis Testing).

Formulation and Plan

Strengths of the Family and Infant

Speak positively and honestly about the strengths of the family. Praise the child for being friendly and cooperative. Compliment the parents for encouraging their baby's autonomy while making sure he or she is safe and for helping their child through the visit. If other siblings are present, compliment them on their strengths as well.

Health Maintenance

Immunizations

If the measles, mumps, and rubella virus vaccine (MMR) is to be given, review the benefits and risks of immunizations with the parent. Confirm that the parents have read the Vaccine Information Statements.* The third dose of inactivated poliovirus vaccine (IPV) may be administered at this visit if it was not given at the 6- or 12-month visit. (Oral poliovirus vaccine [OPV] is not recommended except under special circumstances; if use of OPV is necessary, remind parents that immunosuppressed persons should not be in direct contact with an infant after immunization with OPV.) Give the fourth dose of *Haemophilus influenzae* type b conjugate vaccine if it was not given at the 12-month visit, after discussing the benefits and risks of immunization. Give the third dose of hepatitis B vaccine if it was not given at an earlier visit. Give the fourth dose of DTaP. Give the fourth dose of pneumococcal conjugate vaccine if it was not given at the 12-month visit.

See the current Recommended Childhood Immunization Schedule.

Varicella vaccine may be given at this visit if not previously administered. The Vaccine Information Statements* for diphtheria, tetanus, and pertussis vaccine and for IPV also may be given to the parents in preparation for the immunizations to be given at the next visit.

Anticipatory guidance

◆ Nutrition

Toddlers should eat three meals a day and be supervised by an adult while eating. They should not eat nuts, hard candies, chewing gum, popcorn, hot dogs, grapes, or raisins, which could be aspirated. Toddlers should sit still while eating and swallow all food before leaving the table or high chair. Parents should phase out bottle-feeding if this has not already been done. If foods are warmed in the microwave, stir them thoroughly to even out the temperature. Children should be allowed to use their fingers or a spoon to eat. Table manners are not important. Be aware that toddlers this age typically do not eat much. Vitamins are not necessary if the child is eating fruits or vegetables. Fluoride supplementation may be provided if indicated.

◆ Elimination

Toilet training should be put off until the child is at least 2 years old. Toddlers often become interested in watching their parents using the

---

*Vaccine Information Statements can be obtained from the AAP.

toilet and in observing their own urination or defecation. At that time it is wise to purchase a child-sized "potty" and allow the child to sit on it at will, with diapers in place, as he or she practices training.

◆ **Sleep patterns**

A regular bedtime routine is important. The toddler still needs a nap at least once a day. Even a quiet "rest time" is useful for both parents and child even if the child does not sleep. An object such as a favorite blanket or stuffed animal may be helpful at bedtime. Because some infants will climb out of bed, the crib mattress should be lowered to protect the child from falling.

◆ **Behavior and development**

Children typically seek opportunities for autonomy in eating and playing. Independent eating and exploration should be encouraged. Discuss issues of autonomy and independence with parents, particularly the effect they may have in a particular family. Explain that the child's emerging independence is a part of normal development and not oppositional behavior. Encourage parents to give the toddler immediate and enthusiastic reinforcement for acceptable behavior, delivering more "yes" than "no" messages, and praising good behavior. Spanking is not particularly effective, nor is it a constructive technique of punishment.

To teach the infant appropriate behavior, it is important for parents to set firm and sensible limits, giving a simple message such as "no" when the infant exceeds the limit, and then removing the infant from the potential danger. Advise parents to avoid using toys, candy, or snacks to bribe the child. At this age, it makes sense to distract and redirect the child if the behavior continues after "no" has been heard. Encourage parents to give clear messages appropriate to the child's understanding, and to work together to develop a consistent approach to discipline (see supplement on Effective Discipline, p 225).

Parents should demonstrate how to use and enjoy toys while playing with their child. Household items such as pots, plastic measuring cups, and empty boxes are enjoyed as toys. Parents should encourage imitative behavior (eg, sweeping, dusting, playing with dolls) and provide a safe environment that gives their child the freedom to explore in safety (chasing, dancing, splashing in water, throwing and kicking balls). They will soon enjoy hiding games and representational play (eg, brushing mother's hair, feeding a doll with a spoon).

Parents can stimulate language development by:

❖ Reading books, singing, and talking about what they are seeing and doing.

❖ Naming common animals, objects, and body parts.

❖ Encouraging the toddler to repeat words.

❖ Responding with pleasure to the child's attempts to imitate their words.

❖ Listening to and answering the child's questions.

The toddler will soon learn to climb up and down stairs, to run, to walk backwards, and to kick and throw a ball. These skills are intrinsically reinforcing as they support the child's drive toward increasing autonomy. Children may start to hold and use a large crayon, and they will become increasingly skillful at feeding themselves with a spoon.

◆ **Family relationships**

Temper tantrums are a common phenomenon between 15 and 30 months. Suggestions for their management are discussed in detail in the supplements (p 211).

At this demanding phase of childhood and parenting, it is important that the parents find ways to care for themselves and each other. Parent support groups and educational programs about child development and parenting may be helpful resources.

◆ **Other advice**

Advise parents to limit the amount and to monitor the quality of television programming their child watches; television is not a substitute for interaction with the child.

Encourage parents to begin or maintain their lifetime exercise program, such as walking, running, swimming, or cycling (using a helmet). Emphasize the importance of an environment without cigarette smoke and alcohol and other drugs.

◆ **Injury prevention**

A child with a history of frequent injuries may indicate the possibility of child abuse or neglect.

To prevent trauma:

❖ Review car safety instructions including those about appropriate-sized car seats.

❖ Advise parents to use security gates or lock the doors at stairwells or entrances to potentially hazardous areas, such as the kitchen or basement; window guards should be installed.

❖ Warn parents not to underestimate their child's ability to climb. Chairs should be positioned so that the child is unable to use them to assist in climbing to a dangerously high place.

❖ If a gun is kept in the home, advise parents to store the gun and ammunition in locked, separate locations. (Pediatricians and other child health care professionals are urged to inform parents about the dangers of guns in and outside the home. The AAP recommends that pediatricians incorporate questions about guns into their patient history taking and urge parents who possess guns to remove them, especially handguns, from the home.) Discuss other strategies for violence prevention.

❖ Small children should not be allowed to play with plastic bags or balloons.

❖ Children should always be supervised in or near water (swimming pool, bathtub, lake, ditch, well, uncovered toilet, bucket of water). Knowing how to "swim" does not ensure safety while swimming.

❖ The child should be kept away from hot stoves, space heaters, wall heaters, irons, and fireplaces. Pot handles should be turned toward the back of the stove. Hot liquids on tablecloths or on top of the stove should be closely monitored so they cannot be pulled down.

❖ Parents should not hold or carry the child and hot liquids at the same time. Hot liquids should be kept out of the child's reach during meal preparation.

❖ The hot water heater thermostat should be set at 120°F.

❖ Guard against electrical injuries from cords and outlets by plugging outlets with plastic guards.

❖ Children should wear protective clothing, hats, and sunscreen when going outside.

❖ Reinforce the need for smoke detectors in the home.

Problems and Plans

Review issues discussed and plans to address them (eg, the child resists bedtime or awakens in the middle of the night; recurrent or persistent ear infections).

Closing the Visit

◆ **Have your goals for this visit been met?**

◆ **Are there any other issues you want to discuss? Dealing with new concerns raised at this point may require scheduling a visit sooner than the next routine visit.**

◆ **Set a time for the next visit.**

◆ **Indicate how to contact the office should any concerns arise prior to the next scheduled visit.**

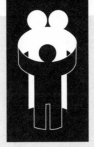

Health Supervision: 18-Month-Old Visit

Health Assessment

Toddlers are delightful, challenging, frustrating, and adorable, all at once. Their development in the areas of language and independence is impressive to behold and demands patience, respect, and consistency from their parents. Cheerful play with a real or an imaginary friend can change in a few seconds to a desperate tantrum. Toddlers really develop "a mind of their own" around this age and may be frustrating when they refuse to do what others ask of them or insist adamantly on doing things their way. When parents see this stubborn independence as evidence of their child's emerging competence and autonomy, they can better enjoy this period with humor and pride.

Interview With Behavioral Observations

Throughout the interview and physical examination, observe the parents' relationship with the child and each other.

Welcoming questions

How is your child doing? How are you doing? What issues or concerns do you want to discuss at this visit?

Check on the status of issues discussed at the previous visit.

Specific questions about the child

◆ Nutrition

Describe the child's usual diet. Does the child still use a bottle? Does your child generally eat three meals a day? How much snacking does your child do between meals? What sorts of snacks? How much milk is your child taking? Who gets together at mealtime? How does mealtime typically go?

◆ Elimination

Is the child showing any interest in the potty? Are diapers ever dry after a nap? What are your plans for toilet training?

◆ Sleep patterns

Where does the child sleep? Does your child fall asleep easily? Does he or she wake up during the night? What do you do then?

◆ Behavior and development

How would you describe your child? Have there been changes in personality or temperament? How does your child express his or her independence or respond to your efforts at teaching or discipline? Has your child had any tantrums? How do you handle them? What do you enjoy most about your child? What aspects of your child's personality do you find challenging? What are some of the new things your baby can do (see Box, Typical Developmental Progress at 18 Months)?

Questions about the family

◆ Family relationships

How does your child get along with you, other adults, and siblings? How do you and other family members handle your child's misbehavior? How does your child respond to your rules and limits? What happens if your child does not do what you want?

Have there been any changes in the family or household constellation? Have there been any recent stresses, illnesses, or crises since the last visit? What are the work schedules of the parents? What child care arrangements have been made?

How often do parents find private time? Who is available to offer support to the parents?

Are there special concerns about other family members, particularly those involving abuse of alcohol or other drugs or the use of excessive punishment or violence? Are there concerns about the methods of discipline used by other family members? Is there a gun in the home?

Typical Developmental Progress at 18 Months

- *gross motor skills:* walks quickly, may run, walks up stairs with one hand held, walks backwards, climbs up onto an adult chair

- *fine motor skills:* eats with a spoon and a fork, stacks blocks, scribbles with crayons

- *cognitive skills:* knows the location of objects that have been hidden, plays at pretend games such as drinking from an empty cup, hugging a toy doll, talking into a toy telephone

- *communication skills:* understands commands, points to body parts on command, may put two words together

- *social skills:* likes to play with other children

Physical Examination With Behavioral Observations

Measurements: *measure and plot percentiles*

- ◆ Height

- ◆ Weight

- ◆ Head circumference

General physical examination

Children typically remain highly resistant to examination at this age. Examining a doll or stuffed animal before examining the child may have a calming effect. To keep the child as comfortable as possible, perform the less invasive procedures first. Observe, then palpate the child. Give the child the opportunity to hold the stethoscope or otoscope before it is used. Give the child as many choices about where and how you will do the examination as possible, eg, on the parent's lap or on the examination table? Which eye should be examined first?

As part of the complete physical examination, make sure to check for tooth eruption, tooth decay, evidence of injuries, proper gait, leg alignment, back alignment, strabismus, and inguinal hernia. Assess hearing and vision.

Observations of behavior and development

Continue to observe the interactions between the caregivers and child. Observe the developmental milestones that were discussed earlier (see Box, Typical Developmental Progress at 18 Months), as well as others insufficiently documented by history.

Observe the child's temperamental characteristics, especially his or her response to constraint or limit setting.

Delays that warrant referral of the child for a full developmental assessment and/or early intervention include not walking, no fine pincer grasp, inability to follow single commands, no understandable words, and persistent, intense stranger anxiety.

Screening Procedures

A hemoglobin or hematocrit should be performed for children at risk. Lead levels should be measured at least annually for children at risk for lead exposure (see Appendix G, Lead Toxicity Screening). If the child or community is at high risk for tuberculosis, a test using purified protein derivative (Mantoux) should be given if not previously done (see Appendix F, Recommendations for Tuberculosis Testing).

Formulation and Plan

Strengths of the Family and Child

Speak positively and honestly about the physical, developmental, and temperamental strengths of the child and the way the parents are managing the child.

Health Maintenance

Immunizations

Ask whether the child had any reactions to the previous immunizations; record information in detail. Parents should have read the Vaccine Information Statements.* Review the benefits and risks of immunizations and answer any questions the parents may have.

Administer the fourth dose of diphtheria, tetanus, and pertussis (DTaP or DTP; DTaP is preferred) vaccine if not given at a previous visit. The third dose of inactivated poliovirus vaccine may be administered at this visit if it was not given at the 6-, 12-, or 15-month visit. (Oral poliovirus vaccine [OPV] is not recommended except under special circumstances; if use of OPV is necessary, remind parents that immunosuppressed persons should not be in direct contact with an infant after immunization with OPV.) Varicella vaccine may be given at this visit if not previously administered. Give the third dose of hepatitis B vaccine if it was not given at an earlier visit.

See the current Recommended Childhood Immunization Schedule.

*Vaccine Information Statements can be obtained from the AAP.

A dose of acetaminophen given in the office or on arrival home with a second dose given 4 hours later reduces the incidence and severity of fever and irritability from the DTaP or DTP immunization.

Anticipatory guidance

◆ Nutrition

Encourage parents to have regular family meals with casual conversation. If the child is growing well, reassure the parents that a decline in appetite has not limited the intake of the essential components of growth. In most circumstances children can decide for themselves how much to eat. Suggest that the parents avoid arguments with their child about food intake. Many children this age have particular and often fickle preferences.

Children should not be allowed to be mobile with food in their mouths. When parents warm foods in the microwave, the foods must be stirred thoroughly to even out the temperature. Discuss weaning from breast-feeding or bottle-feeding if this has not been done. Continue fluoride supplementation if indicated. Vitamins are unnecessary if the diet includes fruits and/or vegetables. Children by this age should be feeding themselves independently and drinking from a cup. Children should not have excessive amounts of fat, sodium, and sugar in their diet.

◆ Elimination

Parents should be encouraged to delay toilet training until the child shows signs of readiness, such as interest in imitating others using the toilet, distress at a soiled diaper, the ability to hold urine for at least 2 hours (eg, diaper is dry after a nap), or a word to signal need to use the toilet. Parents may want to set up a potty chair so that their child can imitate other family members as they use the bathroom. Parents should encourage or offer rewards for success but should not use shame or punishment if the child is not successful. Most children demonstrate readiness for toilet training between 24 to 30 months of age (see supplement on Toilet Training, p 215).

◆ Sleep patterns

Some children continue to take two daytime naps, others may have one midday nap. Even if children resist sleeping during the day, a regular "rest" or "quiet time" should be expected.

Encourage bedtime routines and a regular bedtime. A regular routine of reading to children at bedtime fosters language development and decreases bedtime problems. Frequently encountered sleep problems include resistance to falling asleep, nighttime awakening, and night fears. If these problems disrupt family routines or cause daytime fatigue or irritability in the child or parents, they should be addressed. Parents may be offered the opportunity to discuss the problem at a separate session if time for adequate evaluation and counseling is limited.

◆ **Behavior and development**

Inform parents that children this age rarely share. They enjoy active play such as chase and tag. Symbolic or pretend play tends to be parallel and not interactive. Recommend durable toys (without small parts) that the child can take apart and put back together or use for building (nesting toys, blocks). Children this age are frequently interested in the contents of drawers, cabinets, and wastebaskets!

Reassure the parents that children may still use self-comforting behaviors (such as thumb sucking, masturbation, and attachment to a favorite toy, stuffed animal, or blanket) as ways of handling stress or tension. Inquire about any concerns or fears parents may have regarding these coping strategies.

By 18 months of age, parents need an approach to discipline. Temper tantrums are common. Discourage corporal punishment. This technique is frequently ineffective and communicates that physical force is a legitimate way to solve disagreements (see supplement on Effective Discipline, p 225).

Children this age are rarely distracted or redirected if they really want a forbidden object. Recommend that parents provide clear, simple verbal messages to the child about rules and limits. If the child does not accept the message, then consequences should ensue. The use of natural and logical consequences and of "time-out" is described in the supplement on Effective Discipline, p 225.

Ask parents to consider time-out (brief social isolation) as the discipline measure of choice. Discuss how the parents should use the time-out. Occasionally it may be necessary to use physical reinforcement such as holding the child, moving the object the child has been asked not to touch, or removing the child from a dangerous or forbidden situation. If parents are finding appropriate limit-setting and enforcement of discipline a chal-lenge, a separate session should be arranged for a detailed analysis of the pattern of antecedents, unacceptable behaviors, and consequences after misbehavior.

Remind parents to allow the child to make appropriate choices; autonomy and independence enhance the child's self-confidence. A child who has opportunities to choose activities in some situations may be less resistant to parental restrictions in other situations. Praise the child routinely for good behavior, self-care, and self-expression.

◆ **Injury prevention**

Stair and window safety guards should be in place.

Seat belts or car seats should always be used.

Children must be supervised when playing near a street or driveway.

Children should never be left unattended in a car or alone in the home.

To prevent falls, chairs should not be left in places where the infant can use them to climb to dangerously high places.

Children should be protected from electrical injuries from exposed electrical cords and unprotected outlets.

Guns in the home are a danger to the family. If a gun is kept in the home, advise parents to store the gun and ammunition in locked, separate locations. (Pediatricians and other child health care professionals are urged to inform parents about the dangers of guns in and outside the home. The AAP recommends that pediatricians incorporate questions about guns into their patient history taking and urge parents who possess guns to remove them, especially handguns, from the home.) Discuss other strategies for violence prevention.

Children should always be supervised in or near a swimming pool, bathtub, lake, river, ditch, cesspool, well, or bathroom. Knowing how to "swim" or participating in an infant or toddler aquatic program does not mean the child is safe in or near water.

Advise parents to maintain a tobacco-free and drug-free environment.

Children should not be exposed to direct sunlight without using sunblock.

Reinforce the need for smoke detectors in the home.

Problems and Plans

Review all issues and plans to address them (eg, if another baby is expected, suggest ways to discuss the new baby with their child). Note any positive steps the parents have taken to understand and manage the often challenging behaviors in this new stage.

Closing the Visit

◆ Have your goals for this visit been met?

◆ Are there any other issues you want to discuss? New concerns raised late in the visit may require an additional scheduled visit before the next routine health supervision visit.

◆ Set a time for the next appointment.

◆ Indicate how to contact the office should any concerns arise prior to the next scheduled visit.

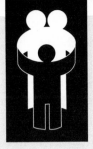

Health Supervision: 2-Year-Old Visit

Health Assessment

Two-year-olds are competent in locomotion. They typically can communicate in short phrases. They remember where parents hid a forbidden object and can coordinate the means to obtain that object. Toddlers explore the limits of acceptable behavior. Parents have the responsibility of teaching appropriate limits while encouraging competence and autonomy.

Interview With Behavioral Observations

It is important to notice throughout the interview and the physical examination how the child and parents interact. Two-year-olds may be independent, exploring the room, sitting in their own chair, answering questions. More often, they rush to a parent when the physician enters and remain on the parent's lap during the examination.

Welcoming questions

How is your family? How are you? What issues do you want to discuss at this visit?

Check on the status of issues addressed at the last visit.

Obtain an interval history regarding illnesses, allergies, accidents, hospitalizations, operations, family changes, or stresses.

Specific questions about the child

◆ Nutrition

What types of food does your child eat? Is your child eating with a spoon and fork? Does your child drink from a cup? How much does your child eat? How much milk does your child drink? How would you describe mealtime in your home?

◆ Elimination

Has your child had any problems urinating or having bowel movements? Has your child begun to show interest in using the toilet (or a potty)? How will you know when your child is ready for toilet training? How do you plan to toilet train?

◆ Sleep patterns

Where does the child sleep (in a bed or a crib)? What is your child's bedtime? Does your child have any problems settling down at bedtime? How do you handle bedtime? Is there a bedtime ritual? If your child wakes up during the night, what happens? What is the schedule of naps?

◆ Development

What are some of the new things your child does? What are your child's favorite toys? What do you like to do with your child? Ask about particular developmental accomplishments (see Box, Typical Developmental Progress at 2 Years).

◆ Behavioral characteristics

How is your child behaving these days? How does your child respond when you say "no"? How often does your child say "no"? How do you interpret your child's refusals?

What are you doing to teach your child to behave appropriately? How does your child respond? How often does your child have temper tantrums? What do you do then?

How does your child respond to being separated from you, such as at the child care center or with baby-sitters?

Describe a typical day. How often does your child spend time with other children and other adults? What does your family typically do together?

Specific questions about the family

How is the family getting along together?

Two-year-old children often challenge parents. How is the communication between the parents? Who else cares for the child? How is that communication?

Typical Developmental Progress at 2 Years

- *gross motor skills:* runs; jumps in place; walks up and down stairs, 2 feet on each step; throws ball overhead
- *fine motor skills:* uses a spoon and fork, opens a door, stacks blocks, draws a vertical line
- *cognitive skills:* early pretend play, remembers place where object is hidden, creates means to accomplish desired end (pulls chair to cabinet, climbs, retrieves hidden object)
- *language skills:* has greater than 50-word vocabulary, speaks several two-word phrases, follows single-step and two-step commands, listens to short stories, uses pronouns
- *social skills:* imitates adults, plays in parallel with other children
- *adaptive skills:* brushes teeth with help, dresses with help, feeds self

Do you have concerns about anyone in the family? Is anyone violent or using excessive punishment? Is anyone dependent on drugs or alcohol? Is anyone depressed? Are there other mental health issues?

Physical Examination With Behavioral Observations

Do not ask a child of this age any questions that may be responded to with "no." A negative response is a 2-year-old's only way of trying to maintain a modicum of control! Simple statements addressed to the child are usually more successful, eg, "Now it's time for me to listen to your heart." For many children the examination may be more easily accomplished on the parent's lap. Where there is truly a choice to be made, it is effective to ask the child for help, eg, "Which ear do you want me to look into first?" Be alert to the presence of physical injuries suggestive of child abuse or neglect.

Measurements: *measure and plot percentiles*

- Height
- Weight
- Head circumference

General physical examination

As part of the complete physical examination, check the child for strabismus. Check the child's hearing (informally).

Observe developmental status

Validate the history provided (see Box, Typical Developmental Progress at 2 Years). Try to observe gross motor, fine motor, and language skills. Observe the child's assistance with undressing or dressing.

Screening Procedures

A hemoglobin or hematocrit should be performed for children at risk. If the child is at high risk for lead poisoning, a blood lead level should be measured (see Box, Lead Toxicity Screening). Determine cholesterol level for high-risk children. Perform a tuberculin test if indicated by high-risk status (see Appendix F, Recommendations for Tuberculosis Testing). Federal Medicaid guidelines require children enrolled in the Medicaid program to have a lead level measurement at 1 and 2 years of age.

Lead Toxicity Screening

Questions to assess risk status for lead poisoning.

Does your child:

* spend time in buildings built before 1950 with peeling or chipping paint, including day care centers, preschools, or the homes of baby-sitters or relatives?

* live in or regularly visit buildings built before 1950 with recent, ongoing, or planned renovation or remodeling?

* have a brother or sister, housemate, or playmate being followed up or treated for lead poisoning?

* frequently come in contact with an adult whose job or hobby involves exposure to lead, such as construction, welding, pottery, or other trades?

* live near an active lead smelter, battery recycling plant, or other industry likely to release lead?

If the answer to any of these questions is YES, the child is considered to be at risk of excessive lead exposure and should be screened with a blood lead test.

For more detailed management, see Appendix G and the AAP policy statement "Screening for Elevated Blood Lead Levels."

Formulation and Plan

Strengths of the Family and Child

Comment on the family's good care of the child, the difficulty of this period of the child's development, and the need for parents and extended family and other supportive persons to work together for the child's development. Note how the child's intrinsic temperament may be interacting with development at this age.

Health Maintenance

Immunizations

Check the child's immunization status and whether the child had any reactions to previous immunizations (see the current Recommended Childhood Immunization Schedule). No immunizations are needed at this visit if they are up-to-date. Hepatitis A vaccine may be required in certain states or regions and for certain high-risk groups; consult your local public health authority.

Anticipatory guidance

◆ **Nutrition**

A healthy diet includes milk, preferably low fat; limits on fat and sugar intake; and fruits and vegetables as snacks. Children should drink no more than 1 quart of milk per day, supplemented by fruit juices if desired. The child should be drinking from a cup or glass exclusively.

Children often develop particular, and changing, food preferences around this age. In most circumstances their choices can be honored without a problem. Multivitamins with fluoride are indicated if the child's diet is consistently inadequate.

◆ **Elimination**

Parents should watch for signs of the child's readiness to use a potty or toilet. It is appropriate to obtain a potty chair around this age, to discuss its purpose, and to allow the child to observe the parents using the toilet. It is preferable (and easier for everyone in the long run) to wait for the child to request the opportunity to imitate its use rather than to insist on it.

◆ **Sleep**

Most children continue to take one nap per day. Even if they sometimes do not sleep, it is wise for parents to insist on a quiet period of rest at a regular time each day.

Children should have a regular hour for bedtime and a predictable bedtime routine. They should be expected to fall asleep in their own bed and to sleep there through the night. Bedtime book reading promotes language development and is often an effective part of a quiet bedtime routine.

◆ **Behavior and development**

Parents should encourage the child's emerging independence and offer choices to the child wherever possible while retaining their authority to make and maintain family rules.

The rate of language development is highly dependent on the family environment. Parents should limit the amount of television and monitor the types of shows their children watch. Parents should try to read a book to their child every day; encourage parents to take their child to the library. Encourage each parent to arrange time one-on-one with each of their children.

Family rules should be established for mealtimes, bedtime, and getting ready in the morning.

Discipline is a frequent concern at this age because of the normally emerging development of autonomy and independence in children. Many conflicts can be avoided by providing children two or three options (choices), each of which is acceptable to the parent(s), eg, "Do you want to wear your sweater or your jacket when you go out to play?" "Do you want orange juice or apple juice?"

Another effective procedure is often to arrange positive outcomes as consequences of acceptable and desirable behaviors. For example, the child receives praise for appropriate play with a friend or obtains dessert for sitting through the meal. In contrast, negative outcomes follow unacceptable behavior. For example, the child cannot go out to play if he hits his playmate. Ideally the parent can combine these approaches. For example, the child can go out to play as soon as he cleans up the mess he created. Introduce parents to "time-out" as an additional discipline strategy, whereby certain defined undesirable actions result in 2 minutes of separation from the family's activities. For example, if a child hits or bites, he must spend 2 minutes in a chair away from the family (see supplement on Effective Discipline, p 225).

Because children this age are exploring the opportunities for independence and its limits, they can be especially challenging for parents. Parents' teamwork is essential in providing the space for children's autonomy to develop while at the same time creating the boundaries necessary to assure children that they will be safe and loved. Parents should be encouraged to find ways to obtain the personal support they need to maintain the physical and emotional energy necessary to this task.

◆ **Injury prevention**

Because of the child's increasing abilities and wish to demonstrate them, parents need to be increasingly watchful for injuries, especially at times of increased family stress.

Medications, cleaning solutions, and household chemicals should be locked in a cabinet because children can climb and reach most areas.

Emphasize the continued need for parents to use appropriate car safety seats.

The hot water heater temperature should be set at 120°F.

Reinforce the need for UV protection.

Smoke alarms should be installed in the home and their operation checked annually.

Guns in the home are a danger to the family. If a gun is kept in the home, advise parents to store the gun and ammunition in locked, separate locations. (Pediatricians and other child health care professionals are urged to inform parents about the dangers of guns in and outside the home. The AAP recommends that pediatricians incorporate questions about guns into their patient history taking and urge parents who possess guns to remove them, especially handguns, from the home.) Discuss other strategies for violence prevention.

Parents need to watch out for potential falls from their child climbing on furniture, window railings, and stairs.

The child should not be fed foods that may be easily aspirated. Children should be watched by an adult at all times while eating. Children should not be allowed to play with a mouth full of food.

Electrical outlets need to be covered with protective "caps."

Parents should not allow the child to play on or around motor vehicles, eg, cars, tractors, or lawn mowers.

Parents should maintain a tobacco-free and drug-free environment.

Teach parents the appropriate use of the emergency medical system (see Appendix E, Preparing Parents for Emergency Medical Services: A Parents' Guide). Inform parents of the importance of providing consent for emergency treatment when they are unavailable.

Reinforce to parents that children are not ready for swimming lessons until after their fourth birthday and that knowing how to "swim" or participating in an infant or toddler aquatic program does not mean the child is safe in or near water.

Problems and Plans

Review any problems or concerns that have been raised during this visit, and clarify plans for each. Offer the opportunity for a specially scheduled visit if parents have concerns about sleep, eating, toilet training, discipline, or other developmental, emotional, or behavioral issues.

Closing the Visit

♦ **Are there any issues or questions that we missed? Have the parents' and the pediatrician's goals been met?**

♦ **Set a time for the next appointment.**

♦ **On the basis of the child and family risk factors, describe those problems that would prompt another visit prior to the next scheduled return.**

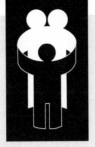

Health Supervision: 3-Year-Old Visit

Health Assessment

Three-year-olds may continue to test limits of acceptable behavior or may be showing increasing acceptance of social limits. Their language skills may exceed cognitive understanding, so that their insights may be quite humorous. An active imagination and imaginary friends are common.

Interview With Behavioral Observations

Children of this age who are developing at the typical rate and who have not had particularly stressful experiences in the physician's office may be able to sit in their own chair or on the examination table, to participate in the discussion, and to build a relationship with the examiner. Initially, compliments to the child may put the child at ease. Then the physician can direct simple questions to the child that are within the child's ability to answer. Throughout the visit, the physician should continue to involve the child.

Observe how the parents and child talk to each other, how much the parent does or says to promote the child's autonomy, how the parent tries to control the child's behavior, how the child responds to the parent, how the child behaves during examination, and how the child utilizes toys or books in the examination room.

Questions to Child

Welcoming questions

Hello. I am Dr_____. How are you? How old are you? Do you go to school? What is your teacher's name? Who is your favorite friend? What things do you like to do best? What is your favorite toy? Would you tell me about your pet? Your new baby sister?

Specific questions

◆ **Nutrition**

What did you eat today for breakfast? What do you like to eat?

Questions to Parent

What has been happening with your child and your family? How would you say things are going for you and your family?

Sometimes parents have some specific issues, concerns, questions, or problems they want to bring to my attention. How about you?

Check on the status of issues at the previous visit.

Since the last visit has your child had an illness, allergies, accidents, or injuries? Has your child been in the hospital? Has your child received any immunizations elsewhere? Have there been any changes in the family?

How is the child's appetite? Does your family observe any dietary restrictions? On a typical day does your child eat a selection of meat, fish, poultry, fruit, vegetables, and grains? How much milk does your child drink? Is your child taking any vitamins or fluoride supplements? How much junk food does your child eat? Is there a family history of elevated cholesterol levels?

Questions to Child

◆ Elimination

Are you wearing a diaper?

◆ Sleep patterns

Where do you sleep? Who else sleeps in that room?

◆ Developmental milestones

What do you like to play? Tell me about your toys.

Do you go to school?

◆ Typical day

What do you like to do with your mother or your father?

Questions to Parent

How is your child doing with toilet training (see supplement on Toilet Training, p 215)? Does your child have any problems having bowel movements? Does your child have any problems urinating or wetting pants?

How well does your child sleep at night? Do you have a bedtime ritual? What helps your child fall asleep? What do you do when your child wakes up during the night? Does your child take a nap (see supplement on Sleep Problems, p 219)?

What are some of your child's new skills? What do you think about your child's development? Ask specific questions (see Box, Typical Developmental Progress at 3 Years, p 103).

Have you considered preschool or nursery school for your child? What would be the advantages? What would be the disadvantages? What opportunities does your child have to play with other 3-year-olds?

What is a typical day like for you and your child? How often do you find time to play and have fun together? How often do you read books with your child?

What are your child care or baby-sitting arrangements?

Questions to Child

- **Temperament**

- **Specific questions about the family**
  Who lives in your house?

Questions to Parent

What do you enjoy most about your child? What do you find most difficult? What are you proud of about your child?

Who does your child remind you of? How does your child react when you say "no"?

How are the relationships at home? Have there been any changes? Any major stresses?

What are your work schedules? How are things at work? Do you have energy left at night?

What are your child care arrangements? How satisfied are you with these arrangements?

How do you discipline your child? Do both parents agree about this? Is anyone excessive in the use of punishment?

Is anyone in the family abusing alcohol or using other drugs? Does anyone have mental health problems?

Physical Examination With Behavioral Observations

Measurements: *measure and plot percentiles*

- Height
- Weight
- Blood pressure

This will probably be the first time the child has had a blood pressure taken, so demonstrate how it will "make the arm feel funny" by rhythmically tightening and loosening your grasp around the child's arm.

The child should be weighed undressed except for wearing underpants or diapers.

General physical examination

As part of the complete physical examination, make sure to perform visual acuity testing, check for strabismus, assess hearing subjectively, evaluate speech, and observe the child's gait, leg alignment, and hip rotation.

Be alert to injuries that could signify child abuse or neglect.

Observations of behavior and development

Validate the information from the interview (see Box, Typical Developmental Progress at 3 Years). Try to initiate conversation with the child. Offer the child the opportunity to copy and draw pictures. Evaluate the child's ability to appreciate pretend play by examining a doll. Also observe the child's behavior, including his or her activity level, ability to cooperate during the physical examination, and sociability.

Screening Procedures

A hemoglobin or hematocrit should be performed for children at risk. Determine levels of lead if the child is at risk (see Appendix G, Lead Toxicity Screening). Obtain a cholesterol level (nonfasting) for high-risk children.

Typical Developmental Progress at 3 Years

- *gross motor skills:* jumps in place, kicks ball, pedals tricycle, walks up stairs with alternating gait
- *fine motor skills:* scribbles, copies a circle, uses utensils, puts on some clothing, can stack at least eight blocks
- *cognitive skills:* participates in pretend play; knows name, age, sex
- *language skills:* speech is at least 75% intelligible; talks in short sentences but may leave out articles, plural markings, or tense markings; asks questions such as "what's that?" and "why?"; understands prepositions and some adjectives
- *social skills:* enjoys interactive play, may be oppositional or destructive, listens to short stories
- *adaptive skills:* undresses, some dressing, progress toward toilet training, self-feeding

Formulation and Plan

Strengths of the Family and Child

Speak positively about the child. "He talks nicely." "How creatively she plays with toys." Acknowledge the caregiving strengths of the parents. "You seem to be very responsive to him." "How well you explain to him what is happening in the exam."

Health Maintenance

Immunizations

Check the immunization status and any reactions to previous immunizations (see Appendix D, Recommended Childhood Immunization Schedule). Perform a tuberculin test if indicated (see Appendix F, Recommendations for Tuberculosis Testing).

Anticipatory guidance

◆ **Nutrition**

Ensure that the child is eating a balanced diet and avoiding junk foods. The child should be feeding himself or herself using utensils. Children should not be fed nuts, hard candies, and chewing gum.

Continue fluoride supplementation if indicated. Parents should encourage children to brush their teeth after meals and before bedtime. Discuss dental care. Parents should schedule a dental appointment for their child.

◆ **Elimination**

Provide information for parents about toilet training if the child is not trained (see supplement on Toilet Training, p 215). By age 3, approximately 90% of children are bowel-trained; 85% of children are dry in the daytime, and 60% to 70% are dry at night. No treatment is necessary for children who are not yet dry at night

◆ **Sleep patterns**

The child may discontinue taking naps. Children may become irritable when they are overtired, particularly after they discontinue naps, and may need help calming down. Switching from a highly active to a more sedentary, restful activity can be helpful before bedtime.

A regular bedtime and bedtime ritual remain important. Parents might consider an earlier bedtime when the child discontinues napping. Occasional night fears are usual (see supplement on Sleep Problems, p 219).

◆ **Development**

Parents should encourage active play with blocks, simple puzzles, beads, and pegs. Children this age enjoy sand and water play, books, and reading. Pretend play, using both toys and household objects, is developing. Passive activities such as watching television should be discouraged.

Language development is facilitated by direct conversation. Children do not learn language in the early stages from television or radio. Parents should provide opportunities for the child to talk about his or her day or other topics of interest to the child. Many children undergo a period of mild speech dysfluency between the ages of 2 and 4 years. This is a transient, self-limited phenomenon.

◆ **Parenting practices**

Each parent should spend some time alone with each child every day.

It is important for the child to explore, show initiative, and communicate. Parents should offer the child choices in appropriate situations. Peanut butter or cheese? Red T-shirt or yellow? This story or that one?

Encourage parents to promote out-of-home experiences for their child, such as nursery school and play groups, as good opportunities to learn and develop social skills such as sharing and taking turns. Discuss the child's ability to be separated from parents and interact with peers. Discuss nursery school selection.

At this age or earlier, children are curious about where babies come from and about the differences between boys and girls. Parents should be prepared to answer these questions honestly, at a level appropriate to the child's understanding and within the boundaries of the question. Children are very honest in expressing their need to know; they will ask questions until their curiosity is satisfied. Advise parents to use correct terms for the genitalia and to understand that the child's sexual curiosity and explorations are normal.

It is important that parents show affection to their child. Children do not understand "tongue-in-cheek" comments and cannot always tell when a parent is joking. Parents should never threaten to leave or abandon their child.

Children should be encouraged to identify with the activities and social roles of their parents. If feasible and culturally appropriate, parents should be discouraged from sharing their bed with their child. Problem-solve how to encourage the child to remain in his or her bed if the parents identify a problem with the child coming to their bed.

Advise parents about discipline. The consequences of unacceptable behavior should be explained to the child. Discipline should be humane, age-appropriate, time limited, and fair (see supplement on Effective Discipline, p 225). Self-discipline and positive sibling relationships need to be encouraged. Parents should encourage their child's independence by allowing some decision making and using "no" sparingly.

Encourage family exercise such as walking, jogging, swimming, or bicycling (with helmet).

Advise parents about the importance of a drug-free and tobacco-free environment.

◆ **Injury prevention**
Children should remain in car seats or booster seats until at least the age of 5. Some booster seats are appropriate for children weighing up to 60 lb.

Doors should be locked to prevent children from falling down steps. A gate should be placed at the top of the stairs.

Children should not play around hot liquids or grease in the kitchen.

Guns in the home are a danger to the family. If a gun is kept in the home, advise parents to store the gun and ammunition in locked, separate locations. (Pediatricians and other child health care professionals are urged to inform parents about the dangers of guns in and outside the home. The AAP recommends that pediatricians incorporate questions about guns into their patient history taking and urge parents who possess guns to remove them, especially handguns, from the home.) Knives should be stored out of the reach of children. Discuss other strategies for violence prevention.

Children should be taught the danger of chasing a ball or a dog into the street, but may not remember such instructions. Children must be closely supervised when near a street.

Children should be advised to be careful around unfamiliar dogs, especially when the dog is eating.

Discuss water safety. This is the earliest age to begin organized group swimming instruction, but parents should be informed that children are not developmentally ready for swimming lessons until after their fourth birthday. Knowing how to "swim" or participating in a toddler aquatic program does not ensure the child's safety in water at this age.

Children should not follow strangers and not allow themselves to be touched by others in ways they don't like.

Medications and poisons should be safely capped and out of sight and reach of children. Syrup of ipecac should be in the home. Remind the parents to call the poison center if the child puts something poisonous in his or her mouth.

Children should not be exposed to direct sunlight without using sunscreen.

◆ **Anticipated siblings**
The room for an expected newborn should be prepared to redefine the child's "space."

Encourage parents to ask friends to bring gifts for the older child, not the newborn.

Schedule the child's next visit prior to the arrival of the baby so full attention can be paid to the older child.

Problems and Plans

Review specific problems and plans for their management (eg, referral to a dentist, follow-up of concern about maternal depression).

Closing the Visit

◆ **Let's review your questions for today. Are you satisfied they have been addressed?**

◆ **Are there other issues you want to discuss? New concerns raised at this point may require a visit sooner than the next routine health supervision visit.**

◆ **Set a time for the next visit.**

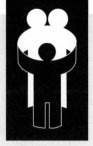

Health Supervision: 4-Year-Old Visit

Health Assessment

Four-year-olds may be quite charming and humorous when their language skills exceed full understanding of the world. Their thinking is egocentric, they believe they are responsible for the moon's moving while they walk or the arguments their parents are having. Some 4-year-olds continue to test limits and have learned ways around their parents' attempts at distraction and discipline.

Interview With Behavioral Observations

*Children this age who have not had stressful experiences in the physician's office should be able to sit in their own chair or on the examination table, participate in the process of providing history, and build a relationship with the examiner. **Address questions first to the child,** then ask the parent for a reaction to the child's answers and for more information. Observe the behavior of the child and parents throughout the history taking and physical examination.*

Parents frequently let their child speak directly with the physician, adding information only when the child is unable to answer or the question is directed to the parent. They may show pleasure in the child's achievements and may encourage independence and expression of feeling. The parents may interact with the child, offering support or setting limits if necessary. Of concern are parents who are depressed or anxious, over-critical and excessively punitive, or indulgent.

Questions to Child

Welcoming questions

How are you? How old are you?
Do you go to school? Where?
What is your school like? What
do you think about school?
Do you want to ask me any
questions today?

Specific questions

◆ **Nutrition**
What do you like to eat?

◆ **Elimination**

◆ **Sleep patterns**
Where do you sleep? What do
you do at night before you go
to sleep?

◆ **Development and behavior**
What sort of things are you
good at doing? Can you draw
a person? Can you get
yourself dressed? Can you
ride a tricycle?

Questions to Parent

How are things going? How is your
child getting along in school or
child care?

What particular issues or concerns
would you like to discuss at this
visit? Check on the status of issues
addressed at the previous visit.

Do you have any concerns about
your child's eating habits, appetite,
or nutrition? Describe a typical
dinner in your home.

Does the child use the toilet for
urinating and having bowel movements both during the day and
at night?

How does your child get to sleep
at night? Where does your child
sleep? Does your child nap? Are
there any concerns about your
child's sleep patterns? Does your
child experience nightmares or
night terrors?

What are some of the things your
child can do that you are proud
of? What skills do you expect of a
4-year-old that your child cannot
perform?

Ask about typical milestones achieved
by a 4-year-old (see Box, Typical
Developmental Progress at 4 Years).

Questions to Child

What is your favorite thing to do in school?

What do you like to do with your mom? With your dad?

◆ **Social relationships**
What are the names of some of your friends? What do you like to do with your friends?

Questions to Parent

How does your child do in preschool? What have you heard from the teachers about your child's development and behavior?

What is your day like? How does your child entertain himself or herself? How much television viewing is permitted? How many videos? How often do you sit with your child and watch television or videos? What other activities do you do with your child?

How do you get along with your child? How does your child get along with friends, peers, siblings, and other adults? At school or in the neighborhood?

Typical Developmental Progress at 4 Years

- *gross motor skills:* pedals tricycle, hops on one foot, balances on one foot, walks up and down stairs with alternating gait
- *fine motor skills:* draws a circle and cross, draws a person with three to six body parts, cuts with scissors
- *cognitive skills:* engages in complex pretend play, may have an imaginary friend, may not differentiate reality from fantasy (may think dreams actually happen), recognizes some of the alphabet
- *language skills:* has extensive vocabulary; uses full sentences of at least six words; fully intelligible to strangers; asks questions with "why," "when"
- *social skills:* engages in interactive pretend play, able to wait turn, able to share, can play board or card game
- *self-help, adaptive skills:* able to put on shirt, pants, socks; able to button and zip; able to brush teeth; uses utensils to eat; toilet trained for both urine and bowel movements

Questions to Child

◆ Temperament

What makes you angry? What do you do when you get angry? What makes you sad? What do you do when you get sad?

◆ Health habits, injury prevention

Do you brush your teeth by yourself? Who puts on your seat belt in the car? What color is your bike helmet?

◆ Specific questions about the family

Who is in your family? What is one thing your family likes to do together? Who takes care of you?

Questions to Parent

How does the child handle anger or frustration or disappointment? How do you handle your child's tantrums, destructiveness, and recklessness? Do you have concerns about your child's level of activity or attention? How does your child comfort himself or herself? Does your child still suck his or her thumb? Do you have any concerns about how your child handles emotions?

Children this age are still at risk for falls. How have you arranged the house to prevent serious falls? What would you do if your child swallowed a poison?

Have there been any changes in the family or household constellation? Have there been any recent stresses, illnesses, or crises since the last visit? What are your work schedules? What child care arrangements have been made? How has the child reacted? How are responsibilities divided at home? How often do you have private time? Are there special concerns about family members, particularly about abuse of alcohol or other drugs or use of excessive punishment or violence? Are there guns in the home? What have you done to ensure that guns cannot be used by your child?

Physical Examination With Behavioral Observations

Continue to observe the interactions between the caregivers and child.

Measurements: *measure and plot percentiles*

- ◆ Height
- ◆ Weight
- ◆ Blood pressure

General physical examination

Reassure the child at the beginning of the physical examination through talking and through touch. The child should be able to discuss the function of the eyes and ears, memories of the last visit, or how to take a bath. It may be possible to perform the examination moving from head to toe. Talking about the physical findings can be instructive to the child and parent and can demystify the office visit as well.

As part of the complete physical examination, make sure to evaluate the child's visual acuity and check for strabismus. Screen the child's hearing, check for dental caries, chronic otitis media with effusion, abdominal mass, and inguinal hernia. Check the child's gait, spine, and upper and lower extremities. Be alert for signs of abuse or neglect.

Observations of behavior and development

Validate historical reports (see Box, Typical Developmental Progress at 4 Years). Observe the child's activity level, attentional abilities, and sociability.

Screening Procedures

A hemoglobin or hematocrit should be performed for children at risk. Lead level should be tested if the child is at risk (see Appendix G, Lead Toxicity Screening). Cholesterol level should be checked for high-risk children. Administer a tuberculin test (PPD) if indicated (see Appendix F, Recommendations for Tuberculosis Testing).

Formulation and Plan

Strengths of the Family and Child

Speak positively and honestly about the physical, developmental, and temperamental strengths of the child. "Look at how well he answers my questions!"

Health Maintenance

Immunizations

Inquire about whether the child had any reactions to the previous immunizations; record information in detail. Parents should read the Vaccine Information Statements,* if not previously done. Review the benefits and risks of immunizations, and answer any questions the parents may have. Develop a method to obtain consent for vaccination if a person other than the parent brings the child to the visit.

Before the child enters school (4 to 6 years of age), administer the fifth dose of diphtheria, tetanus, and pertussis (DTaP or DTP; DTaP is preferred) vaccine, the fourth dose of inactivated poliovirus vaccine, and the second dose of measles, mumps, and rubella virus vaccine. (Oral poliovirus vaccine [OPV] is not recommended except under special circumstances; if use of OPV is necessary, remind parents that immunosuppressed persons should not be in direct contact with an infant after immunization with OPV.) Hepatitis A vaccine may be required in certain states or regions and for certain high-risk groups; consult your local public health authority.

See the current Recommended Childhood Immunization Schedule.

A dose of acetaminophen given to the child in the office or on arrival home and a second dose given 4 hours later may reduce the incidence and severity of fever and irritability from the DTaP or DTP vaccination.

Anticipatory guidance

◆ Nutrition

Reassure parents whose child has a poor appetite or limited food preference if the child's growth rate has been normal. This can be illustrated for optimal effect by reviewing the child's growth chart with the parent. The child's poor appetite and finicky food preferences may persist. Suggest that parents offer small portions first, with second helpings if the child wants more food. Parents should make an effort to create a pleasant

---

*Vaccine Information Statements can be obtained from the AAP.

atmosphere at mealtime with table conversation that includes opportunities for the child to participate. The child's diet should avoid excessive amounts of fat, sodium, and sugar.

Children should have dental visits twice per year.

◆ Elimination

Provide advice regarding toilet training if the child has not completed the training. Sometimes regression occurs in toilet training as the child assumes greater responsibility for determining the need to go to the toilet. By age 4, 95% of children are bowel trained, 90% are dry during the day, and 75% are dry at night. Because nighttime wetting is common at this age, no specific interventions are warranted.

◆ Sleep patterns

Encourage children to sleep in their own beds if compatible with the family's culture. Parents should create a calm bedtime ritual that could include reading or telling stories to promote language development and prereading skills. Nightmares and night terrors are common at this age. Discuss the parents' approach to a sleep disturbance. Family stresses should be evaluated in children with sleep disturbances.

◆ Social relationships

Parents should try to provide opportunities for the child to play with peers, either in the neighborhood or at school. Children can accept some chores such as setting the table for meals and helping clean afterwards. They can keep a bargain. They enjoy pretend play and mastering difficult situations. They may play games with rules, but they often interpret rules as optional rather than required, and applicable only when the rules are to their advantage.

Reassure parents that masturbation is quite common as a part of self-discovery and learning to associate genital stimulation with pleasant sensations. Masturbation is normal if it is private and not highly preferred over most other activities. It should involve stimulation only of the external genitalia and leave no signs or symptoms.

Sexual play between young children also occurs regularly and is generally simple, noninvasive, brief, and mutually pleasing. Preschool children may frequently try to touch the breasts or genitalia of their parents.

◆ Good parenting practices

Parents should establish a balance between the child's need for independence and the need to educate their child about social rules and limits on behavior. Children can demonstrate independence by dressing and feeding themselves. Discipline at this age is challenging. It is recommended that parents reprimand children for bad behavior in private, providing appropriate and clearly stated limits and consequences if rules are broken. Many 4-year-olds require supervision to ensure that rules are followed. Nagging and idle threats by parents are ineffective. It is important that parents follow through with stated consequences when rules are broken. Social isolation (time-out) remains an effective conse-quence for many children; time-outs can be increased to 5 minutes. The positive effects of praise are often more powerful behavior modifiers than negative reinforcement (such comments as "I really like it when you let your friends play with your toys," or "Thank you for waiting quietly while your father and I talked").

Nursery school or child care experiences should be considered for children who have not experienced out-of-home care. This experience prepares the child for the social expectations of a classroom and the required separation from parents. Active play in noncompetitive settings should be encouraged.

Advise parents to establish family exercise programs such as walking, jogging, riding a bike (with a helmet), or swimming.

◆ Injury prevention
Preschool children need close supervision in the home and neighborhood. Toys should be age-appropriate and safe. Sharp corners on furniture should be padded, or the furniture should be removed from the child's play area. Electrical tools, firearms, matches, and poisons must remain out of the reach of children.

Falls are still common. Parents should consider gates on stairs and window guards. Burns are also common. Children should play away from hot liquids and grease in the kitchen.

Children require supervision when riding a tricycle or playing near the street. Bicycle helmets must be worn while riding when they learn to ride a bicycle.

Children and adults should always wear car seat belts or use a car seat properly.

Parents should be reminded to call the poison center if the child puts something poisonous in his or her mouth. Syrup of ipecac should be in the home.

Children must be supervised near water. Children should be watched by a responsible adult who can swim. Because most children are now ready developmentally for swimming lessons, instruction enhances the child's safety.

Reinforce the need for smoke detectors in the home.

In case of a fire in the home, the family should have a plan of escape.

The child should be instructed not to talk to or accept food from strangers.

Children should be instructed to tell their parents if they are touched in a manner that seems inappropriate or unpleasant.

Children should be careful around strange dogs.

Guns in the home are a danger to the family. If a gun is kept in the home, advise parents to store the gun and ammunition in locked, separate locations. (Pediatricians and other child health care professionals are urged to inform parents about the dangers of guns in and outside the home. The AAP recommends that pediatricians incorporate questions about guns into their patient history taking and urge parents who possess guns to remove them, especially handguns, from the home.) Discuss other strategies for violence prevention.

At this age, children can be taught to dial "911" by themselves or to call their local emergency ambulance service or county emergency medical service.

Inform parents of the importance of providing consent for emergency treatment when they are unavailable.

Reinforce the need for UV protection.

Problems and Plans

Review specific problems discussed and plans for their management (eg, if the child has limited exposure to other children, encourage the parents to set up play groups with other families; if the child always has the television volume loud and shouts, suggest that the child undergo a hearing test).

Closing the Visit

◆ **Have your goals for this visit been met?**

◆ **Are there any issues we missed? New concerns raised late in the visit may require an additional scheduled visit before the next routine health supervision visit.**

◆ **Set a time for the next appointment.**

◆ **Indicate what concerns would warrant a return prior to the next scheduled visit. Remind the parents how to contact the office to set up such an appointment.**

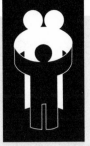

Preface to
School-Age Children

The health supervision of school-age children should reflect their physical, psychological, and social development. Although physical growth during the school years is not as rapid as during infancy or adolescence, size and physical ability form important parts of a child's developing self-concept. Changes in cognitive development and social skills contribute to the child's understanding and interaction with the world.

Most children associate visits to the physician with receiving immunizations. Fortunately, since most health supervision visits in school-age children do not require immunizations, this apprehension should be alleviated at the onset of the visit. Other children may feel they are expected to "perform" during the visit; this anxiety may be diminished with appropriate preparation and parental support.

What distinguishes health supervision visits in this age group is the importance of dealing with the child as an increasingly independent individual. During the school years children become able to make decisions that influence their health. Lifelong patterns of health behavior often begin at this time. Health supervision visits are opportunities to help children become competent decision makers and to feel a sense of responsibility about their own health. These goals are promoted when physicians engage children actively in discussions about their health and well-being.

Begin each visit with an open-ended greeting to both the parent and the child. Children do their best when they are not anxious. Talking to children directly and allowing them to answer simple questions helps build the child's confidence and enhance rapport. Comments about clothing, upcoming holidays, and birthdays are often good ways of putting children at ease.

In contrast to adults, children this age should initially be asked simple, direct questions such as their age or the names of their friends. It is common for children to feel somewhat anxious when questioned; if they respond to your initial questions, respond positively and continue to ask questions. If the child does not respond, you may ask a few more questions, but proceed with interviewing the parents, being sure not to convey displeasure toward the child. Many children will become more expressive as the interview and examination progress.

Involving the child during the visit also helps to develop a therapeutic alliance. Physicians and parents need to let children know that their views are valued. Children can provide considerable information about their friends, daily activities, and health habits and are more likely to respond spontaneously to questions that have not already been answered by the parents. Listening to the child allows further insight into the child's personality, emotive style, and cognitive abilities. Communication with the child does not need to be limited to verbal exchanges. Asking younger children to draw pictures or older children to write down a class schedule can enhance communication and be very informative. In addition, direct communication demonstrates your interest in the child as an individual and establishes a sense of trust and confidentiality.

During this period, school achievement and social relationships become critical for children's psychological and social growth. Time spent with friends either on their own or in organized activities supervised by adults, television viewing, activities with parents, and chores form, in descending order, the daily time allocation of children when outside school. Through all these activities, children develop values that play an important role in future behavior. Because many adults other than parents now spend a considerable amount of time with children, they become important sources of information. A report card or conversation with a teacher or other supervisor can be enlightening.

To parallel the increasing responsibility that is given to the child during the office visit, the child can be given increasing responsibility for decisions about personal health, diet, exercise, and illness and can be encouraged to meet with the physician independently for a part of each visit. During illness, the child may be encouraged to report a change of symptoms, although the parent may be in charge of controlling important health behaviors. Many problematic health behaviors, or their precursors, emerge as early as age 5. Because physicians are viewed by children as important adults, they have the potential to be a powerful influence on important health behaviors in a few well-spent moments during office visits.

Parent and Child Guides to Pediatric Visits may be helpful as an adjunct to the health supervision visit (see Appendix C). For some children and adults, the opportunity to organize their observations and questions prior to their meeting with the physician leads to greater efficiency and satisfaction with the encounter.

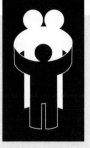

Health Supervision: 5-Year-Old Visit

Health Assessment

Five years old marks a transition from preschool to school age. Children may remain egocentric in their thinking but may be asked to follow rules of the classroom. Children may also remain highly imaginative as they learn new skills and facts at school.

Interview With Behavioral Observations

When a child is 5 or 6 years old, some pediatricians may choose to spend a few minutes talking with the child alone during the visit. The child can be called into the examination room alone before the parents join them. At each subsequent visit, the proportion of time with the child alone can gradually increase.

Children this age should be able to participate actively in providing a description of their activities, diet, school, and peers. It is preferable to begin the interview by speaking directly to the child, looking to the parents for agreement, elaboration, and further description.

Children are frequently cheerful and talkative during the examination. They enjoy demonstrating their new skills. They can perform tasks such as drawing with a reasonable attention span. They relate well with adults and accept limits set by either their parents or the physician. They know the difference between reality and fantasy. Be concerned if the child seems withdrawn or excessively fearful, irritable, overly sensitive, aggressive, or impulsive.

Questions to Child

Welcoming questions

How are you? What should we talk about today? Do you have any questions for me about your body or health?

How old are you? Where do you live? Where do you go to school? How many brothers and sisters do you have?

Have you been sick since I saw you last?

Specific questions

◆ **Nutrition**

What do you like to eat? What are your favorite snacks?

◆ **Toileting**

Do you have any problems with bowel movements ("poop") or urinating ("pee")? If the child is unresponsive, ask the parent what toileting terms are used at home.

Questions to Parent

How is your child doing? How is your family doing? How are things going for you?

Check on the status of issues addressed at the previous visit.

Since the last visit, has your child had any illnesses, accidents, injuries, hospitalizations, or operations?

Have there been any changes in the family?

How does your child eat? Are there disagreements between you and your child about what or when your child eats? Do you have any questions about what your child should be eating? Do you have concerns about your child's weight?

Does your child use the toilet consistently during the day? Does your child wet the bed at night? Does he or she have bowel movements outside of the toilet or soil his or her underpants?

Questions to Child

◆ **Sleep patterns**

What is your bedtime? Do you nap during the day?

◆ **School**

What grade are you in? Who is your teacher? How do you like your teacher? What do you like most about school? What do you not like about school? Who is your favorite friend?

◆ **Development and behavior**

Do you have a tricycle? Can you ride a bicycle with training wheels? Can you write your name?

Questions to Parent

Does your child have any difficulties going to bed? Does your child have nightmares or wake up in the middle of the night? How does your child wake up in the morning? Does your child nap?

What was school like for you when you were a child? What do you think school will be like for your child?

How has the transition to school worked for each of you thus far? How do you feel your child is doing? What feedback have you had from the school? What does your child tell you about what he or she does in school?

Can your child skip and ride a bicycle with training wheels?

Does your child get dressed independently? Can your child fasten small buttons and zippers? Can your child tie his shoes?

Can your child tell a simple story or retell a fairy tale? How well does your child express himself or herself verbally? Is the language understandable by all children and adults? What letters of the alphabet can your child recognize? Write? How high can your child count? What numbers does your child recognize?

How long can your child sit to hear a story? Watch a video or television show (see Box, Typical Developmental Progress at 5 Years, p 125)?

Questions to Child

What do you like to play with? What do you like to do with your friends? What shows do you watch on television?

What would you do if someone grabbed a toy you were playing with? What do you feel when your mom or dad says "no"?

◆ **Injury prevention**

Who wears a seat belt in your car? Do you always wear a seat belt? Do you wear a helmet when you ride your bike? Have you taken swimming lessons? What would you do if there was a fire in your house? What would you do if a strange man came up to you after school and offered you a ride home?

◆ **Your family**

What things does your family like to do together? What do you do with your dad? Your mom? Your brothers or sisters? What is special about your family? What would you like to be different about your family?

Questions to Parent

What is a typical day like for your child? Do friends from school come to your home after school and on weekends? What child care arrangements have you made for after school hours? What are your family's rules about television?

How would you describe your child? What makes you proud of your child? How would you describe your child's activity level? Perseverance? Ability to adapt to change? How does your child respond to frustration, disappointment, or change?

What are the family rules about seat belts? Bike helmets? Swimming? Do you have a gun at home? Where and how is it stored? Are you aware of the risks of guns for small children? Are poisons, electric tools, and flammable chemicals locked up? Have you discussed how your child should treat strangers? Do you have smoke detectors in your home? Have you discussed with other family members what to do in case of fire? What are your rules about playing in the neighborhood? Does your child follow the rules?

What do you like to do with your child? What kinds of activities do you do as a family? Have there been any particular stresses in the family recently? Do you anticipate any? How does your child get along with you? Your other children? Does anyone in the family abuse alcohol or other drugs? Has anyone in the family ever been hurt intentionally?

Questions to Child

♦ **Discipline**

What happens in your house if your dad or mom doesn't approve of something you're doing? What are your chores around the house? What happens if you don't do your chores? What do you do when you get angry? When did your mom or dad get angry with you?

Questions to Parent

How do you manage to get your child to do what you want? What do you do if your child doesn't respond? What are your discipline techniques? How are they working? How often do you punish your child? How? Do you ever worry your discipline is too lenient or too severe?

Typical Developmental Progress at 5 Years

- ♦ *gross motor skills:* balances on one foot, hops, skips, able to climb up to examination table
- ♦ *dexterity:* able to tie a knot, has mature pencil grasp, draws a person with at least six body parts, prints some letters and numbers, able to copy squares and triangles
- ♦ *language or communication skills:* tells a simple story using full sentences, appropriate tenses, pronouns; counts to 10; names at least four colors; has good articulation
- ♦ *social skills:* follows simple directions, able to listen and attend, undresses and dresses with minimal assistance

Physical Examination With Behavioral Observations

Respect the child's increasing modesty.

Measurements: *measure and plot percentiles*

- ♦ Height
- ♦ Weight
- ♦ Blood pressure

General physical examination

As part of the complete physical examination, evaluate the child's hearing and visual acuity. Check for strabismus.

Observations of behavior and development

Notice the child's interaction with each parent.

◆ Does the parent attend to the child and listen to what the child has to say?

◆ Does the parent give praise, approval, and support?

◆ Does the parent allow the child to communicate with you directly, or does the parent interfere in your interaction with the child?

◆ Does the parent seem proud of the child's abilities and accomplishments, or impatient and critical?

◆ Does the parent appear to provide clear expectations for the child's behavior, or does the parent seem rigid and punitive?

◆ Does the parent have realistic expectations for the child's age and developmental abilities?

◆ Does the child communicate with respect and in a friendly way with his or her parents?

◆ Is the child oppositional or provocative?

Notice the child's interactions with you.

◆ Is the child friendly and cooperative?

◆ Is the child mute or excessively shy?

◆ Is the child's language understandable? Are the child's syntax, vocabulary, grammar, and content appropriate for his or her age?

◆ Does the child appear angry or depressed?

◆ Does the child follow your directions?

◆ Is the child destructive?

◆ What is the child's level of concentration, attention, or activity?

◆ Does the child seem proud to describe his or her friendships, activities, and emerging skills?

Developmental milestones

(see Box, Typical Developmental Progress at 5 Years)

Screening Procedures

A hemoglobin or hematocrit should be performed for children at risk. A screening urinalysis should be done. Perform a tuberculin test as indicated (see Appendix F, Recommendations for Tuberculosis Testing). Obtain a blood lead level if indicated (see Appendix G, Lead Toxicity Screening). Cholesterol level should be obtained for high-risk children. Children at risk should be screened for sexually transmitted diseases.

Formulation and Plan

Strengths of the Family and Child

Comment on the family's care of the child and the child's developmental progress. Comment on the child's temperament and, if appropriate, how it will help the child adopt to the new tasks of the coming year.

Health Maintenance

Immunizations

Inquire about whether the child had any reactions to the previous immunizations; record information in detail. Parents should read the Vaccine Information Statements,* if not previously read. Review the benefits and risks of immunizations and answer any questions the parents may have. Develop a method to obtain consent in case a person other than the parent brings the child to the visit.

Before the child enters school (4 to 6 years of age), administer the fifth dose of diphtheria, tetanus, and pertussis (DTaP or DTP; DTaP is preferred) vaccine, the fourth dose of inactivated poliovirus vaccine, and the second dose of measles, mumps, and rubella virus vaccine as indicated by local regulation. (Oral poliovirus vaccine [OPV] is not recommended except under special circumstances; if use of OPV is necessary, remind parents that immunosuppressed persons should not be in direct contact with an infant after immunization with OPV.) Hepatitis A vaccine may be required in certain states or regions and for certain high-risk groups; consult your local public health authority.

See current Recommended Childhood Immunization Schedule.

A dose of acetaminophen given to the child in the office or on arrival home and a second dose given 4 hours later may reduce the incidence and severity of fever and irritability from the DTaP or DTP vaccination.

*Vaccine Information Statements can be obtained from the AAP.

Anticipatory guidance

◆ **Injury prevention**

Discuss safety practices for storing guns, poisons, and electric tools in the home; car safety belts and bike helmets; pedestrian and bicycle safety practices; water safety; fire safety (alarms, safe escapes); and dealing with strangers. (Pediatricians and other child health care professionals are urged to inform parents about the dangers of guns in and outside the home. The AAP recommends that pediatricians incorporate questions about guns into their patient history taking and urge parents who possess guns to remove them, especially handguns, from the home.) Discourage skateboarding and in-line skating unless proper protective equipment is used, including a helmet and elbow, wrist, and knee pads. Reinforce the need for UV protection. Counsel the parents about violence prevention.

◆ **Preventive health practices**

Encourage children to eat a healthy diet; discourage eating "junk food"; encourage pleasant family mealtime experiences; fat, sugar, and sodium intake should be limited in the diet.

Promote regular physical activity for the family.

Children should brush their teeth twice a day and have routine dental visits.

Adequate sleep is necessary; children should sleep in their own beds and have a bedtime routine.

◆ **Active parenting practices**

Parents need to spend time playing with their children every day.

Parents should encourage their child's increasing independence and autonomy and help the child practice making good age-appropriate decisions.

Parents should encourage their children to interact with other children.

Encourage parents to show affection and pride in each child's special strengths and use praise liberally.

Remind parents to demonstrate interest in their child's activities and achievements.

Encourage the child to interact with grandparents and other adults.

Future independent reading should be encouraged by recommending that families read together and by suggesting a particular favorite book.

Mechanisms for solving family problems (eg, family meetings) should be in place.

Television viewing should be limited and monitored.

Encourage parents to discuss sexuality with their child as appropriate to the child's age and interest.

Problems and Plans

Review any problems and clarify plans for their management. It may be helpful to write down a summary for parents to take home (eg, if the child is difficult to wake in the morning, set an earlier bedtime as a routine).

Closing the Visit

◆ **Have any issues or questions been missed?**

◆ **Have the goals of the pediatrician and parents been met? Unmet needs may require arranging a visit before the next regular visit.**

◆ **Set time and purpose for next scheduled appointment.**

◆ **Indicate how to contact the office should any concerns arise prior to the next scheduled visit.**

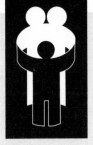

Health Supervision: 6-Year-Old Visit

Health Assessment

Most 6-year-old children have entered elementary school. They are expected to observe classroom rules, regulate their attention and behavior, and learn academic material. Children who succeed in the school environment typically feel self-confident. Children who have difficulties with social or academic demands may feel inferior or depressed.

Interview With Behavioral Observations

During this visit, talk to the child as much as possible. Ask the child questions first, then ask the parent for a response to the child's answers or for more information. The visit should feel like a discussion with the family. To improve the flow of information, you may decide to offer anticipatory guidance during the interview as topics come up. For example, advise parents about a healthy diet while you are asking how the child is eating; remind the child to use the helmet after he tells you he rides his bicycle every afternoon.

Questions to Child

Welcoming questions

How old are you? Where do you go to school? What grade are you in? How are you getting along?

Is there anything special you want to tell me about today? What questions would you like to ask me? Do you have any worries you need to talk about now?

Check on the status of issues addressed at the previous visit.

Since I saw you last, have you been sick? Have you had any type of injury (broken bones, stitches), allergies, immunizations ("shots") given elsewhere, or have you gone to the hospital?

Specific questions

◆ **Nutrition**

How have you been eating? How does your mother think you are eating?

Questions to Parent

From your perspective, how are things going for your child and family since your last visit? What issues, questions, or concerns would you like us to discuss at this visit?

Check on the status of issues addressed at the previous visit.

Since I saw you last, has your child been sick? Has your child had any type of trauma (broken bones, stitches), allergies, immunizations given elsewhere, or hospital stay? Have there been any family crises or stresses (illness, unemployment, death, separation, divorce, or remarriage)?

How is your child's appetite? What does your child eat for proteins (meat, poultry, fish, or beans)? Does your child eat some fruits and vegetables every day? How much milk does your child drink? Does your child take any vitamins? Tell me about mealtime in your home. Is the television turned on during meals? How does that affect the interactions of the family? How do you determine if your child has had enough to eat? How much junk food does your child eat? Is there a family history of a cholesterol problem?

Questions to Child

◆ Elimination

Do you have a bowel movement every day? Is it hard or soft? Does it hurt? Do you ever soil your pants? Is urinating comfortable? How many times do you have to go to the bathroom during school? How often do you have to get up at night to urinate? Do you ever wet your bed or pants?

◆ Sleep patterns

What is your bedtime? What time do you wake up? How do you sleep?

◆ School

What do you think about school? What is your teacher like? Do you like your teacher? What is your favorite thing to do at school? Your worst? Do you like your school?

◆ Development and behavior

Can you ride a bicycle?

Can you print your name? Tie your shoes?

Show me your left hand.

Please draw a picture of a child like you.

Questions to Parent

Some children at this age have problems with wetting, bedwetting, or soiling. Does your child have any of these problems? Do you have any concerns about constipation or diarrhea?

How does your child fall asleep? Alone in bed? Bedtime ritual? How often does your child wake up in the middle of the night? How often does the child have to be awakened in the morning?

What are your expectations for your child at school? How has the transition to school worked for each of you? What feedback have you had from the school?

How would you evaluate your child's abilities in sports? Does he or she move smoothly? Can he or she pedal a two-wheel bicycle?

How are your child's abilities to draw and write? Does your child have any trouble understanding long commands or complex sentences?

Can your child tell a story about a recent event? How do you feel about your child's readiness to learn how to read? To do math?

Questions to Child

What do you do after school? Who takes care of you then?

Who is your favorite friend at school? How often do you see your friend after school or on weekends? Who is your best friend in the neighborhood?

What makes you angry? What do you do when you get angry? What makes you sad? What do you do when you feel sad?

◆ **Injury prevention, risk assessment**

Who wears a seat belt in your car? Do you always wear a seat belt? Do you wear a helmet when you ride your bicycle? Have you taken swimming lessons? What would you do if there were a fire in your home? What would you do if a strange man came up to you after school and offered you a ride home? Where do you play outside?

Questions to Parent

Do friends from school come to the house after school and on weekends? What child care arrangements have been made for after-school hours? How are the arrangements working out? What are your family's rules about watching television? Do you watch television together?

How does your child get along with peers? Do you notice any problems with making friends? Keeping friends?

What are some things about your child that make you especially proud? What is your child's usual mood? How does your child handle frustrations? Separations? Do you have any concerns about your child's behavior? What are some reasons you might get angry or annoyed with your child?

What are the family rules about seat belts? Bicycle helmets? Swimming? Do you have a gun at home? Where and how is it stored? Are you aware of the risks of guns for small children? Are poisons, electric tools, and flammable chemicals locked up? Have you discussed with your child how to respond to strangers? Do you have smoke detectors in your home? Have you discussed a plan of escape from your home in case of fire?

Does your child play outside? How well does your child follow street safety rules?

Questions to Child

◆ **Your family**

What things do you like to do with your family? What are some things you like to do with your dad? Your mom? Your brothers or sisters? What would you like to be different about your family?

What happens in your house if your dad or mom doesn't approve of something you're doing? Are your mom and dad pretty fair for the most part? What are your chores around the house?

Questions to Parent

What do you like to do with your child? What kinds of activities do you do as a family? Have there been any particular stresses in the family recently? Are any anticipated? Does anyone in the family abuse alcohol or other drugs? Has anyone in the family ever been hurt intentionally? How well do people communicate in your family?

How do you manage to get your child to do what you want? What do you do if your child doesn't respond? What method of discipline do you use? How is it working? What do you do if your child continues to misbehave?

Physical Examination With Behavioral Observations

Respect the child's modesty.

Measurements: *measure and plot percentiles*

◆ Height

◆ Weight

◆ Blood pressure

General physical examination

As part of the complete physical examination, check the child's gait and spine on forward bending. Perform a visual acuity test. Test the child's hearing if it has not been tested at school or if hearing or speech problems or language delay is suspected.

Validate the developmental history. The child should be able to skip, draw a picture of a child with 8 to 12 or more features, recount a personal story about a recent event, follow a three- to four-part command, recognize the alphabet, and count to 20.

Consider whether the child is friendly, interested, comfortable, cooperative, open, verbal, secure, and trusting — or shy, anxious, highly distractible, and unable to accept limits.

Screening Procedures

Check cholesterol level for high-risk children. Perform a tuberculin test if indicated (see Appendix F, Recommendations for Tuberculosis Testing).

Formulation and Plan

Strengths of the Family and Child

Comment positively about the strengths of the parents and child. "I'm really glad you are limiting the television time and getting out for a family walk each day," or "I'm so happy that you have made friends in your new school."

Health Maintenance

Immunizations

Inquire about whether the child had any reactions to the previous immunizations. When the child is between the ages of 4 and 6, administer the fifth dose of diphtheria, tetanus, and pertussis vaccine and the fourth dose of poliovirus vaccine (see the current Recommended Childhood Immunization Schedule). Administer the second dose of measles, mumps, and rubella (MMR) vaccine if not yet given. Hepatitis A vaccine may be required in certain states or regions and for certain high-risk groups; consult your local public health authority. Have the parents read the Vaccine Information Statements* and answer any questions they may have.

Anticipatory guidance

Address comments and suggestions to children whenever appropriate, requesting support and attention from parents as well.

◆ **Nutrition**
Advise the parent and child to eat a well-balanced diet that avoids excessive amounts of junk food. Consider the need for vitamin, fluoride, iron, or calcium supplement. Encourage regular physical activity.

*Vaccine Information Statements can be obtained from the AAP.

◆ Dental care

Children need to brush their teeth twice a day, including at bedtime, and floss daily. Regular dental visits should be scheduled.

◆ Good parenting practices

Parents should spend active time with their child daily and praise and encourage their child's activities. Remind parents to show affection and pride in each child's special strengths and use praise liberally. Remind parents that they are their child's role model in terms of activities, values, attitudes, and morality.

Parents should reinforce their child's independence and self-responsibility. Rules should be established to be followed at home such as bedtime rituals, television watching, chores such as setting the table or keeping the child's bedroom neat.

Parents should encourage reading and other hobbies; the child can obtain a library card, and the family can make routine trips to the public library. Consider enrolling the child in community youth sports or encouraging family activities such as biking, running, and swimming. If the child is involved in organized sports, parents should ensure that the coach emphasizes learning and play rather than competition and winning.

It is important to maintain a tobacco-free, drug-free environment.

◆ Injury prevention

Children should wear appropriate helmets and protective gear while bicycling, skating, and in-line skating. Children should learn to swim. To avoid sunburn, parents should limit the child's exposure or use sunscreen. Adults and children should always use seat belts. This is the earliest age at which children are developmentally ready to ride on a snowmobile. They should not operate a snowmobile until at least age 16. A safety helmet should be worn if riding a snowmobile.

Parents must decide which streets the child may walk alone; review crossing streets at corners, looking both ways, using traffic lights. Parents should observe the child before he or she walks alone. Remind the child not to talk to or get in cars with strangers.

Guns in the home are a danger to the family. If a gun is kept in the home, advise parents to store the gun and ammunition in locked, separate locations. (Pediatricians and other child health care professionals are urged to inform parents about the dangers of guns in and outside the home. The AAP recommends that pediatricians incorporate questions about guns into their patient history taking and urge parents who possess guns to remove them, especially handguns, from the home.) Counsel the parents about violence prevention.

Ask parents to make sure smoke detectors are installed and working. Matches should not be within the reach of children. Good adult supervision should be arranged when parents are away.

Problems and Plans

Review any problems and clarify plans for their management (eg, if a hearing deficit is suspected, refer the child for audiometry; if a grandparent has died, discuss how the family can help the child).

Closing the Visit

♦ **Did we discuss everything each of you wanted to cover at today's visit?**

♦ **Are there other issues you need to discuss?**

♦ **Set a time for the next visit.**

♦ **Indicate specific issues (physical, psychological, or school-related) that warrant a return appointment prior to the next scheduled visit.**

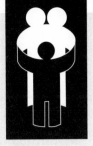

Health Supervision: 8-Year-Old Visit

Health Assessment

Middle childhood was once considered the latency period. However, we know now that this period is marked by considerable development in academic skills, physical abilities (especially in sports), social interactions, and emotional regulation. School success and home life are both important for the maintenance of self-esteem.

Interview With Behavioral Observations

Children this age should be able to provide a considerable amount of history and should build a positive relationship with the examiner. Look toward the parent after the child answers your questions for agreement and elaboration. Observe the behavior of the child and parents throughout the history and physical examination. Parents should provide praise, approval, support, and attention. The parents should encourage the child's independence, including friendships and interests outside the home. The parents should also take pride in the child's abilities and achievements.

It may be appropriate to deal with concerns and questions as they arise in the interview.

Questions to Child

Welcoming questions

How are you? How are things going? What would you like to discuss about your health?

Check on the status of issues addressed at the previous visit.

Specific questions

◆ Nutrition
How is your appetite? What do you like to eat for breakfast? Dinner? Snack?

◆ Elimination
Do you have any problems using the bathroom?

◆ Sleep patterns
What time do you go to bed? How many hours do you sleep on a school night? On weekends? Do you have nightmares?

◆ School
Where do you go to school? What subjects do you like? What subjects do you dislike? What do you think about your grades? Are there other issues you would like to discuss about school?

Questions to Parent

What issues, questions, or concerns do you have regarding your child's health and well-being? Have there been any changes in your child's health status? Has your child had any illnesses, hospitalizations, or operations since the last visit? Is your child taking any medications?

Do you have any concerns about your child's eating, appetite, or nutrition?

Do you have any concerns about toileting, bedwetting, or soiling?

Do you have any concerns about sleep patterns?

Do you have any questions or concerns about your child's school? How are your child's grades? Reading skills? Handwriting? Math? How is your child's behavior and attendance at school? What did you learn at the parent-teacher conference?

Questions to Child

◆ **Development and behavior**

What do you like to do for fun? What activities do you participate in at school or after school? Sports? Clubs? Hobbies? Read? How many hours each day do you watch television?

Who are your friends? What do you like to do with your friends? How do you and your friends get along? What problems do you have with friends, classmates, or adults?

How would you describe yourself? Active? Happy? Sad? Friendly? Shy? What accomplishments are you proud of? Who can you talk to if you're feeling sad? What about mad?

◆ **Health and safety habits**

What protective gear do you wear when playing sports? Do you wear a helmet when riding your bike?

Questions to Parent

What are your expectations for your child in terms of sports and extracurricular activities? How would you rate your child's commitment and skills in these activities? How many hours of television a day do you permit your child to watch? Do you have rules? Who watches your child after school?

How does your child get along with friends, peers, and adults? At school? In the neighborhood?

What's your child like? How does your child compare with other family members? How often does your child seem extremely sad or angry? How does your child express and deal with these feelings?

What are your rules for playing around water (lake, stream, pool, or ocean)? Is an adult always present? Does your child consistently wear a helmet when riding a bicycle? Do you have firearms in your home? Where are they stored?

Questions to Child

♦ **Your family**
How are you getting along with your siblings? How are you getting along with your parents?

Questions to Parent

How could communication in the family be improved? Have there been any changes in the family or household constellation or any recent stresses, illnesses, or crises since the last visit? What is your work schedule? What other responsibilities do you have at home? Do you feel you have enough private time? Do you have any special concerns about family members (particularly about abuse of alcohol and other drugs or excessive use of punishment or violence)?

Physical Examination With Behavioral Observations

Measurements: *measure and plot percentiles*

♦ Height

♦ Weight

♦ Blood pressure

General physical examination

You may want to begin the physical examination by examining the child's hands to reassure the child. Observe the child's speech and language. The child should have total mastery of all sounds in his or her first language, have mature sentence structure, and be able to recount personal anecdotes or stories.

As part of the complete physical examination, test the child's visual acuity. Perform objective testing of the child's hearing. Note early signs of puberty, including skin changes, body sweat/odor. Observe the child's activity level, attentional abilities, and sociability.

Screening Procedures

Check cholesterol level for high-risk children. Perform a tuberculin test if indicated (see Appendix F, Recommendations for Tuberculosis Testing).

Formulation and Plan

Strengths of the Family and Child

Speak positively and honestly about the physical, developmental, and temperamental strengths of the child and about the parent-child interaction.

Health Maintenance

Immunizations

Check the status of routine immunizations (see the current Recommended Childhood Immunization Schedule).

Anticipatory guidance

Address comments and suggestions to the child whenever appropriate.

- ◆ **Nutrition**
  Advise the child directly about good health habits including eating a well-balanced diet and avoiding junk food. Encourage the child to eat breakfast daily. Children can maintain appropriate weight through a combination of sensible dietary intake and regular physical activity and should not be "on a diet."

  Children should brush their teeth at least twice a day, including once at bedtime, and floss daily. Regular dental visits should be scheduled twice per year.

- ◆ **Sleep patterns**
  Provide guidelines for adequate sleep. Children age 8 typically sleep 9 to 12 hours per night.

- ◆ **Pubertal development**
  Observe and discuss the child's pubertal development and encourage the parent to discuss and consult with the pediatrician.

- ◆ **Good parenting practices**
  Discuss establishing a balance between the child's need for independence and the need for children to learn the household rules and consequences if rules are broken. Recommend regular family interactions around meals and/or other activities.

Parents serve as role models in terms of behavior, attitudes, and morality. At the same time, parents should encourage peer play and activities, including sports, clubs, and camps that are outside the home. Other opportunities to encourage independence and responsibility would be to help the child obtain a library card or to give an allowance. Recommend fair, understandable rules about chores, television watching, outside activities, homework, and bedtime. It is important that parents follow through with stated consequences when rules are broken. Loss of privileges (grounding) becomes an effective method of discipline when children have planned recreational activities and opportunities to visit with friends (see supplement on Effective Discipline, p 225).

Encourage parents to maintain active communication with the child. An interest in the child's daily school activities and encouragement for the child's other activities promote a sense of accomplishment and self-esteem. Some children who do not want to participate in a team sport can be encouraged to consider an individual sport such as swimming, dance, or gymnastics. The child must feel free to confide fears and worries to the parents without fear of punishment.

Ensure that parents have made appropriate child care arrangements for when they are not at home. They should know where their child is at all times. Discuss the importance of maintaining a drug-free and tobacco-free environment.

Consider discussing puberty, especially for girls.

◆ **Injury prevention**
Discuss the child's participation in team sports. Parents should ensure that safety is a priority and that the goal is fun and not winning. Trampoline use by children is discouraged unless supervised by a trained professional.

Children should wear appropriate helmets and protective padding while bicycling, skating, and skateboarding. Adults and children should always wear seat belts. Children should be taught an escape plan in case of fire in the home. Reinforce the need for UV protection.

Children can be advised to learn rescue breathing.

Guns in the home are a danger to the family. If a gun is kept in the home, advise parents to store the gun and ammunition in locked, separate locations. (Pediatricians and other child health care professionals are urged to inform parents about the dangers of guns in and outside the home. The AAP recommends that pediatricians incorporate questions about guns into their patient history taking and urge parents who possess guns to remove them, especially handguns, from the home.) Counsel the parents about violence prevention.

Reinforce the need for smoke detectors in the home.

Problems and Plans

Review other issues and plans to address each of them (eg, if the child does not excel in sports, focus on other activities such as model building, stamp collecting, dance, music, and chess; if the child is overweight, review diet and exercise).

Closing the Visit

◆ **Have your goals for this visit been met?**

◆ **Have any issues been missed?**

◆ **Set a time for the next appointment.**

◆ **Indicate how to contact the office should any concerns arise prior to the next scheduled visit. Discuss interest and willingness to aid in the assessment or treatment of psychosocial, developmental, or school problems that might arise.**

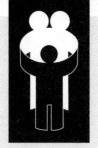

Health Supervision: 10- and 11-Year-Old Visit

Health Assessment

Children this age may be in middle childhood or may have entered early adolescence. In early adolescence, children become focused on body image. Their peer group becomes an increasingly important influence on style, attitudes, and values. They may begin risk-taking activities such as smoking cigarettes or drinking alcohol. Parents may be unprepared for many of these changes.

Interview With Behavioral Observations

If it is comfortable for the child, take some time to communicate alone or utilize private time with the child during the physical examination. Parents must also be consulted to verify and expand some of the child's answers.

Explain confidentiality, including its inclusions and exclusions.

Questions to Child

Welcoming questions

How have you been? How is everything going for you? What issues or concerns would you like to discuss today?

Specific questions

◆ Nutrition

What do you think is meant by a well-balanced diet? Is your diet well balanced?

◆ Elimination

How frequent are your bowel movements? Do you experience pain or burning with urination? Are bowel movements painful, hard, or very loose?

◆ Pubertal development

For girls: Have you heard about menstruation? What do you expect when you begin menstruating? Do you have any discomfort in your breasts?

For boys: Have you heard of wet dreams? What is your understanding about them? What do you know about erections?

Questions to Parent

In general, how are things going? What has happened since we last met? Are you concerned about poor performance or attendance at school? Headaches, stomachaches? Lack of friends? Eating and sleeping problems? Disobedience, aggressive or destructive behaviors? Effeminate or tomboyish mannerisms? Smoking, use of alcohol or other drugs?

How would you characterize your child's diet? How much junk food does your child eat? What are the sources of calcium and iron in your child's diet? Does your child take vitamins? Is there a history of elevated cholesterol levels in your family? How much fat does your child eat? Does your child have regular dental checkups?

Do you have concerns about your child's toileting?

Have you explained menstruation/wet dreams to your child?

Questions to Child

◆ **Sleep patterns**

How have you been sleeping? How do you feel when you wake up?

◆ **School**

What grade are you in? What school do you attend? How are you doing in school? What is your best subject? Your worst? How do you get along with the teacher(s)? How do you get along with your classmates?

◆ **Activities**

What do you do after school and on weekends? What sports do you play? Do you have hobbies? How much television do you watch each day? How much time do you spend reading?

◆ **Social relationships**

How do you get along with your parents? What do you like to do together as a family? What happens if you don't follow the rules?

How are you getting along with the children in your neighborhood? Where do you spend your time after school? How often do you play with friends?

Questions to Parent

Estimate how much sleep your child gets. Do you have concerns about how much sleep your child gets?

How is your child progressing? What is your understanding of problems in school? How would you characterize your child's level of ability? How is your child's ability to pay attention? Does your child act out? How is the teacher addressing the problem? How does your child get along with the other children?

What are the household rules regarding homework? What are the rules regarding watching television?

How are you getting along as a family? What are the most enjoyable activities you do together? What activities are most likely to cause friction or problems? How often does your family interact together with the television off? How would you describe dinner and dinnertime conversation?

Are you comfortable with your after-school child care arrangements?

What do you think about your child's friends?

Questions to Child

◆ **Emotional well-being**
Tell me one thing about yourself that you're proud about. What makes you feel worried, sad, or mad? How often do you feel this way? Who do you talk to when you feel this way? What else do you do?

◆ **Health habits and risk assessment**
Are any of your friends smoking cigarettes, drinking alcohol, or using other drugs? How would you handle an invitation to join them in any of these behaviors?

Have you noticed any changes in your body? What have your parents explained to you about the changes you may go through? What have you learned at school? What are your questions?

Questions to Parent

What are some of the things that make you especially proud of your child? What concerns you? Have you ever been concerned that your child is depressed or anxious? How do you help your child when he or she is sad or angry?

Have you been concerned that your child is using cigarettes or alcohol or other drugs?

Physical Examination With Behavioral Observations

Depending on the level of physical development of the child and on your sense of the child needing to talk to you alone, offer the child the privacy of having the parent wait outside while you do the examination. Make sure to respect the child's modesty.

Measurements: *measure and plot percentiles*

◆ Height

◆ Weight

◆ Blood pressure

General physical examination

As part of the complete physical examination, make sure to include an assessment for scoliosis, Tanner stage, and examination of genitalia.

Perform objective assessments of vision and hearing unless performed at school and the results are normal and verifiable. Perform a pelvic examination on girls and conduct screening for sexually transmitted diseases as indicated. A chaperone may be needed during the physical examination.

Observations of behavior

At this age, the child may be expected to display self-confidence with a sense of mastery and pride in school and extracurricular activities, make friends and participate in group activities, understand and comply with most rules at home and at school, and assume reasonable responsibility for his or her own health, school work, and chores.

Be concerned if the child lacks self-confidence; is distressed with his or her physical appearance or ability to function (eg, the child feels too small, too fat, or too clumsy); is unable to make or keep friends; is sad, joyless, or depressed; is doing poorly at school; or is aggressive or unable to abide by rules.

Screening Procedures

A hematocrit or hemoglobin determination in menstruating females should be done annually, and urine dipstick analysis for leukocytes should be done at least once between 11 and 21 years of age but annually for sexually active children and adolescents. Perform a cholesterol test for high-risk children. Perform a tuberculosis skin test (Mantoux) if indicated (see Appendix F, Recommendations for Tuberculosis Testing).

Formulation and Plan

Strengths of the Child and Family

Reinforce the strengths of the child and parents with comments such as "I'm so pleased that you are making good progress with your math tutor," or "It's so good that despite your busy schedules, you have arranged a family sit-down dinner five nights a week."

Health Maintenance

Immunizations

Review the child's immunization status. Make sure to use and document the use of the appropriate Vaccine Information Statements.* Administer a tetanus-diphtheria (Td) booster. Hepatitis B; measles, mumps, and rubella (MMR); and varicella immunization may be indicated. Make sure to schedule subsequent doses of hepatitis B vaccine (see the current Recommended Childhood Immunization Schedule). The second dose of MMR vaccine is recommended routinely at 4 to 6 years of age but may be administered during any visit, provided at least 4 weeks have elapsed since receipt of the first dose and that both doses are administered beginning at or after 12 months of age. Those who have not previously received the second dose should complete the schedule by the 11- to 12-year-old visit. Hepatitis A vaccine may be required in certain states or regions and for certain high-risk groups; consult your local public health authority.

Anticipatory guidance

◆ Good health habits and risk reduction

Advise children to eat a well-balanced diet, eat breakfast before school, avoid eating excessive amounts of junk food, and get regular physical exercise. When children exercise and participate in sports, maintenance of adequate hydration is important, especially in warmer climates and when there is increased humidity, solar radiation, or air temperature. Family members should pursue lifelong exercises such as walking, jogging, cycling, and swimming. The age of 10 is a prime year for sports competition. Year-round participation in multiple sports may reduce injuries from overuse of the same muscle groups. Strength training is appropriate under proper supervision.

Children should brush their teeth at least twice a day, including once at bedtime, and floss regularly.

Children should avoid smoking cigarettes, drinking alcohol, and using illicit drugs.

For children who are in puberty or interested in sexual activity, encourage abstinence. Remind children to report sexual advances of any kind. Encourage parents to consult with pediatrician about the child's pubertal development.

*Vaccine Information Statements can be obtained from the AAP.

◆ **Injury prevention**
Car seat belts must always be used. Other appropriate protective gear, such as bicycle helmets and helmets and protective padding for skateboarding and in-line skating, should be worn. Trampoline use should be discouraged.

Guns in the home are a danger to the family. If a gun is kept in the home, advise parents to store the gun and ammunition in locked, separate locations. (Pediatricians and other child health care professionals are urged to inform parents about the dangers of guns in and outside the home. The AAP recommends that pediatricians incorporate questions about guns into their patient history taking and urge parents who possess guns to remove them, especially handguns, from the home.) Discuss violence prevention with child and parents.

Parents need to arrange adult supervision for their child when they are away.

Water activities and the use of power tools must be supervised.

Children at this age should not operate personal watercraft. When participating in water sports, a child should wear a US Coast Guard–approved personal flotation device.

Children should be protected from sunburn.

Reinforce the need for smoke detectors in the home.

◆ **Good parenting practices**
It is beneficial for children to observe affection and interest from their parents, and for parents to spend active time with them daily. They should communicate with the child about daily activities and praise good work. Rules and expectations should be discussed, clarified, and enforced.

Parents should limit their child's television viewing and supervise the types of programs that are watched; it is helpful for parents to watch and discuss programs with their child.

Parents should gradually provide opportunities for age-appropriate decision making and independence. One option is giving the child an allowance or offering job opportunities so that the child can learn to manage modest amounts of money.

Parents should prepare girls for menarche. They should answer their child's questions about sex comfortably. If there are questions they can't answer, they should find the answer with their child. Various books are available that may assist parents with these discussions, and pediatricians can help parents answer questions.

Problems and Plans

Clearly state any problems identified during the visit and the plan for their management. It may be useful to help with problem-solving efforts through compromise (eg, if the parent and child have been angry with each other over putting things away, suggest that they compromise by having the child pick up after himself or herself in every room in the house except his or her own room).

Closing the Visit

♦ **Have your goals been met?**

♦ **Set a time for the next appointment.**

♦ **Indicate how to contact the office should any concerns arise prior to the next scheduled visit. It is appropriate to suggest that the child could call independently if he or she has a question to discuss with the physician or nurse (give the child a card with the office telephone number).**

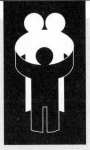

Preface to the Adolescent and Young Adult Years

Health supervision visits during the adolescent years differ significantly from those in infancy and later childhood. As children mature, they become much more interested in and capable of assuming responsibility for their own health needs. They also become keenly aware, inquisitive, and concerned about body changes and functions. The pediatrician may acknowledge these developments by increasing the involvement of the adolescent in each visit and by renegotiating the relationship between the physician and the adolescent's family to emphasize the opportunity for adolescent-initiated visits and confidential discussions without a parent present. In addition, the length of time required for each visit and the content of the visit will change from visits in previous years. These changes should be discussed prospectively with the adolescent and his or her parents.

Parent and Child Guides to Pediatric Visits may be helpful as an adjunct to the health supervision visit (see Appendix C). For some children and adults, the opportunity to organize their observations and questions prior to their meeting leads to greater efficiency and satisfaction with the encounter.

The psychosocial content of the interview during adolescence should reflect recognition of the developmental tasks faced during this time and include questions to determine the adolescent's developing mastery of these tasks. During these years, psychological and social independence from the family is increasing, sexual identity is more firmly established, and plans for the future with regard to education and employment are developing.

This gradual process occurs over 8 to 10 years and is divided into stages defined largely by the adolescent's psychological development (which often mirrors physical development). These developmental stages are *early adolescence,* the period of rapidly changing physical and sexual development (puberty) and psychological changes that reflect separation from authority figures; *middle adolescence,* associated with intense psychological and physical involvement with peers; and *late adolescence,* characterized by emancipation from parents and preparation for a career and more intimate relationships.

It is important to recognize that an adolescent's social and/or emotional life can greatly influence his or her physical health. Conversely, adolescents with chronic illnesses may have significant psychosocial concerns. Risk-taking behaviors are more commonly observed in adolescents than in younger children and should be addressed during the interview, examination, and formulation. Throughout adolescence, it is important to assess the risk for suicide.

The way in which the clinician asks questions about issues such as sexual behavior and drug use depends on the developmental stage of the adolescent, the clinical situation, and the physician's style of interviewing. Adolescents are likely to respond more honestly and less anxiously if the questions fit appropriately into the context of the interview; the reason for each question is obvious; the physician is straightforward, comfortable, and nonjudgmental; and the adolescent's desire for privacy is respected. Questions about sexual behavior or the need for contraception can easily be brought up at several points, eg, during discussions of relationships, menstruation, nocturnal emissions, or sex education. It is important not to assume heterosexuality, but to provide an opportunity for open discussion about all questions about sexual attractions and behavior.

The topic of drugs can be broached in the course of discussing peer influences, pressures in school, or general health habits. The physician may then move comfortably from a discussion of tobacco and alcohol to one concerning marijuana and other illicit substances. In addition to discussing drugs and alcohol, the adolescent should be observed for signs of substance abuse.

The physical examination, which is best done without the parent present unless the adolescent insists otherwise, is an important psychotherapeutic tool when used to reassure the adolescent about the normalcy of his or her body. During the examination the interview should continue and emphasize questions about body concerns. A dialogue can be encouraged by a statement such as: "During the examination, it would be a convenient time to bring up questions that you may have about your body and its changes — things that didn't come to mind before." The physician, rather than waiting until the physical examination is completed, should give the adolescent appropriate reassurance as the examination proceeds: "Your heart is fine...your blood pressure is normal...your breasts are normal."

Parental needs for physician advice and support remain high during adolescence. The physician should educate parents about stages of adolescent development and provide opportunities for parents to ask questions and clarify their concerns. **Policies regarding confidentiality must be stated clearly to both parents and adolescents and strictly adhered to.** Because there may be times when breaking confidentiality would be lifesaving, such circumstances should be discussed with the parents and the adolescent.

The content of the physical examination should reflect the possibility of the increased involvement of adolescents in athletic activities. Physicians should assess overall health, muscle strength, and joint flexibility to best counsel the young athlete on the prevention of injuries. In addition, self-examination techniques of the breasts and genitalia should be demonstrated during the examination. A pelvic examination is indicated for females who are sexually active or who complain of menstrual disorders.

The ability of the pediatrician to recognize and acknowledge the adolescent's developing intellectual and physical maturity should be evident in his or her approach to the health supervision visits during these years. During late adolescence, the transition to care by a nonpediatrician provider can be facilitated through discussions between the pediatrician and the adolescent.

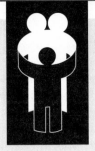

Health Supervision: 12- and 13-Year-Old Visit

Health Assessment

Early adolescence typically begins between 10 and 14 years of age. It is characterized by rapid physical growth and sexual development (puberty). It is a time of beginning independence and separation from parents; the child becomes unwilling to participate in some family activities, concentrates on peer relationships, casts off old patterns of behavior, and challenges parental authority. Early adolescents may show a continuation of concrete thinking or may show early signs of the ability to think abstractly. Adolescents in this stage show an increased concern with their developing body and often compare themselves with peers to assess their own normality. Heterosexual and homosexual experimentation are common. Early adolescence may be a particularly trying time for both adolescents and parents.

Interview With Behavioral Observations

It is usually advisable to create opportunities to interview the child and the parent together and the child alone. In front of the parents pledge confidentiality to the child, eg, "Anything that you tell me that you want me to keep private, I will not tell your parents; I will keep your confidence completely, unless you tell me that you are going to hurt yourself or hurt someone else." It may be appropriate for you to speak with the parents alone also, while maintaining confidentiality. One option is to speak with both the adolescent and parent and then have the parent wait in another area while you talk further with the adolescent; when you leave the room while the adolescent undresses, you have the opportunity to talk with the parent. After the adolescent has been examined, invite the parent to join you so the formulation can be done with everyone present.

The health care professional should explicitly discuss the rules of confidentiality with both the adolescent and parents early in the interview. The adolescent's confidentiality should be respected unless information is revealed that indicates that the adolescent or another person is at serious risk. Health care professionals can alert the adolescent, prior to any discussion, that they will encourage the adolescent to discuss any problems with their parents, although the final decision about the content and timing of communication with the parents is the adolescent's.

Questions to Child

Welcoming questions

How is everything going? How have you been? What issues or concerns do you want to discuss at this visit?

Check on the status of issues addressed at the previous visit.

Specific questions

◆ **Interval history**

Since your last visit, have you had any significant illnesses, hospitalizations, allergies, injury, or immunizations?

◆ **Nutrition**

What do you typically eat for breakfast, lunch, and dinner? What do you eat for snacks? Do you take iron supplements or vitamins? Are you interested in gaining or losing weight?

How often do you see a dentist? When was your last dental visit?

◆ **Elimination**

How frequent are your bowel movements? What is their consistency? Do you have any discomfort when you have a stool? Do you have problems with soiling? How frequently do you urinate? Do you experience a need to suddenly urinate, painful urination, or wetting?

◆ **Pubertal development**

For girls: Has the onset of menses occurred? Do you understand what it is about? How frequent are your periods? Do you experience discomfort? What do you use to protect your clothing when you have your period?

Questions to Parent

I suspect you have some issues or concerns now that your child is an adolescent.

Have there been any significant family stresses (moves, parental marital changes, family member illness or death, changes in household composition, parental job loss)?

How satisfied are you with your child's eating habits? Do you have any concerns about your child's weight? Do you have a family history of cholesterol problems?

Do you have any questions about your child's adolescent sexual development? Have you discussed menstruation and sexuality with your daughter? How can I help you with this?

161

Questions to Child

For boys: Have you experienced nocturnal emissions? Are you aware that this is completely normal?

◆ **Sleep patterns**
What is your usual bedtime? What time do you awaken? Do you think you get enough sleep? Is it hard to get up in the morning?

◆ **School**
How is school going? How are your grades? Tell me about some of the things you do best at school. How do you get along with your classmates?

◆ **Typical activities**
What do you do for fun? Do you participate in sports, clubs, or religious activities? What are your hobbies?

◆ **Social relationships**
How are things going at home? What does your family enjoy doing together? How do you feel about the rules in your house? What privileges do you have regarding money, allowance, curfew, visits from friends, choosing clothes, wearing makeup, using the telephone? Do you think they are appropriate? What responsibilities do you have? Do you think they are appropriate? What happens if you don't fulfill your responsibilities?

Questions to Parent

Have you discussed sexuality and sexual function with your son? How did it go? How can I facilitate communication between you and your son?

Do you have concerns about your child's sleep patterns?

From your vantage point, how is school going for your child this year? What do you think about your child's grades? How often does your child miss school? Have you spoken to your child's teachers recently?

How are you getting along with your child? How do the child and siblings get along? How does your child get along with other children? What do you think about your child's friends? What do you like to do as a family? How are family rules made and enforced in your home? What privileges does your child have? What is your household policy about watching television? How could communication in your family be improved? Does your child confide in you?

Questions to Child

How is it for you to make friends? Are you attracted to anyone special? Who? What are your thoughts about dating? Are your friends starting to have sex? What are your thoughts about having sex?

◆ **Emotional well-being**

Who do you talk to when you are worried or scared? What are some of the things you worry about? Your health? Your development? Is there anyone who annoys you a lot? What makes you sad or angry? What do you do when you are really angry at your parents? Have you ever considered running away? Have you ever thought about suicide?

What kinds of changes would you like to see in yourself? What would you like to do better? What would you like to change about your life? Are there any suggestions you would like me to make to your parents?

◆ **Health habits and risk assessment**

Do you have any friends who smoke cigarettes or drink alcohol or use other drugs? Have you tried any of these? How often do you use them? How much do you use?

Where did you learn most of what you know about sex? From your parents, friends, or classes at school? Let's review

Questions to Parent

What are some of the things that make you especially proud of your child? Has anything displeased you? What has worried you? What is your child's usual mood and attitude? Is your child happy? Is it easy or hard for your child to express feelings? What about for you (or others at home)?

Have you ever thought your child might be drinking alcohol or using other drugs?

What are your concerns about your child's sexual behavior or sexual orientation? Do you have any questions for me?

Questions to Child	Questions to Parent
what you know about body and sexual changes, nocturnal emissions, masturbation, erections, ejaculations, menstruation, petting, and intercourse? Are you attracted to boys, girls, or both? What are your thoughts about having sexual intercourse? Do you know the risks and how you can lower your risks? What questions would you like to ask me?	
Do you participate in sports? What have you heard about supplements or medications to build muscle? Have you tried any of these? How do you gain or maintain weight for the sport?	

Physical Examination With Behavioral Observations

During the examination give the adolescent the option of being examined alone or accompanied by a parent. Ask, "Do you want your parent to stay with us or to wait outside while I talk with you further and examine you?" It is good to be alone with the child, both to talk further and for examination, but do not push the child if he or she seems uncomfortable being examined alone. Each situation varies — that of a mother with a prepubertal boy is different from that of a father with a daughter in puberty. Respect the patient's modesty.

Measurements

Measure and plot the child's height and weight; you may want to plot the child's height on a velocity curve. *Look for a growth spurt in girls between 11 and 13½ years of age and in boys between 13 and 15½ years of age.* Obtain the child's blood pressure.

General physical examination

As part of the complete physical examination, make sure to include an evaluation of the Tanner stage. Look for physiologic gynecomastia in boys and asymmetric breast development in girls. Check the child for goiter.

Instruct the child in self-examination of the breasts or testicles. Examine external genitalia and perform a pelvic examination if the child is sexually active. Screen the child for scoliosis with an upright and forward bending test. Assess the child's vision and hearing. Evaluate the skin for acne. Assess athletic girls and girls planning active involvement in sports for disordered eating, menstrual dysfunction, and decreased bone mineral density. Assess athletic boys and boys planning active involvement in sports for disordered eating.

Observations of behavior and development

Assess the adolescent's interaction skills by listening to what the adolescent says and by observation. Is the adolescent friendly, interested, comfortable, cooperative, confident, open, secure, and trusting? Or tense, shy, suspicious, guarded, silent, angry, anxious, highly distractible, or provocative?

Screening Procedures

A hemoglobin or hematocrit determination should be done for menstruating girls. Perform blood lipid screening if indicated by family history or by risk factors, such as obesity, hypertension, smoking, or diabetes.

In sexually active adolescents, perform screening for chlamydia, gonococci, and syphilis; perform a Papanicolaou smear (in girls) and HIV testing if requested or if the adolescent is at high risk. Perform a tuberculin skin test (Mantoux) if indicated (see Appendix F, Recommendations for Tuberculosis Testing).

A urine dipstick analysis for leukocytes should be done at least once between 11 and 21 years of age but annually for sexually active children and adolescents.

Formulation and Plan

Strengths of the Child and Family

Reinforce the strengths of the child, eg, "I'm really happy that you have thought about what we talked about and feel you are able to withstand peer pressure about the use of alcohol and other drugs." Reinforce the strengths of the parents, eg, "You seem to be doing an effective job structuring appropriate expectations and enforcing them."

Health Maintenance

Immunizations

Administer the second dose of the measles, mumps, and rubella (MMR) vaccination if it has not yet been given. Provide and discuss the Vaccine Information Statements* with the parents. Menstruating girls must be advised not to become pregnant for 3 months after rubella immunization. A hepatitis B immunization series may be started if not previously given, with the second and third doses given at 1 month and 6 months, respectively. Varicella vaccine may be given if the adolescent has not had natural chickenpox or the vaccine (see the current Recommended Childhood Immunization Schedule). Hepatitis A vaccine may be required in certain states or regions and for certain high-risk groups; consult your local public health authority.

Anticipatory Guidance

Many issues of anticipatory guidance, such as diet, maturation, and sex education, may be discussed as they come up during the history taking or the physical examination.

- ◆ **Injury prevention**

    To minimize the risk of injury when riding bicycles, children and adults should always wear helmets.

    Seat belts in cars should always be worn.

    Adolescents should never accept a ride in a car if the driver has been drinking. Adolescents must not accept rides from strangers or hitchhike.

    Children younger than 16 years should not drive or ride on all-terrain vehicles.

    Everyone should take precautions to avoid sunburn.

    Adolescents need to avoid locations where tobacco smoke is present.

    Adolescents need to be taught to resolve interpersonal conflicts without violence.

    Guns in the home are a danger to the family. If a gun is kept in the home, advise parents to store the gun and ammunition in locked, separate locations. (Pediatricians and other child health care professionals are urged to inform parents about the dangers of guns in and outside the home. The AAP recommends that pediatricians incorporate questions about guns into their patient history taking and urge parents who possess guns to remove them, especially handguns, from the home.) Discuss violence prevention with child and parents.

*Vaccine Information Statements can be obtained from the AAP.

For activities in which there is a risk of eye injury, protective eyewear should be worn.

Discuss the need for UV protection with the child and parent.

Reinforce the need for smoke detectors in the home.

◆ **Good health habits and risk reduction**

Adolescents should engage regularly in physical activities, such as walking, running, swimming, tennis, and bike riding. Provide advice on sports conditioning, fluids, weight training, and protective equipment. If there is a family history of heart attacks at early ages and high cholesterol levels, perform cholesterol screening — if the adolescent's cholesterol level is elevated, review diet, weight maintenance, exercise, and avoidance of other cardiac risks such as smoking.

Weight can be maintained through a good diet, sensible eating habits, and routine exercise. Discourage crash diets, medications, laxatives, or forced emesis. Encourage avoidance of nicotine, alcohol, and stimulant drugs such as anabolic steroids.

Adolescents should be aware of the importance of adequate calcium intake. Inform them about calcium-containing foods.

Encourage sexual abstinence. Emphasize the child's right to refuse sexual contact and to report sexual abuse. If the adolescent seems uneasy or fearful about peer pressure to become sexually active or wishes to discontinue sexual activity, offer support and specific suggestions for managing vulnerable situations. If the adolescent is sexually active, emphasize the importance of a sense of responsibility with regard to oneself and one's sexual partner. Offer advice about contraception and discuss the reproductive implications of sexual activity and the prevention of sexually transmitted diseases.

◆ **Good parenting practices**

Remind parents to:

Establish procedures for making and enforcing family rules.

Allow the adolescent to make age-appropriate decisions and selections (eg, choosing clothes).

Spend time with their adolescent and maintain comfortable communication.

Make arrangements for the adolescent's supervision when they are absent from home.

Praise and encourage the adolescent's activities at home and outside the home, attend events in which the child is a participant, contribute to the child's self-esteem, show affection, and respect the child's privacy.

Supervise potentially hazardous activities (eg, the use of power tools, firearms, participation in water sports).

Continue to play a role in their child's sex education, perhaps with the aid of books recommended by the physician, followed by dialogues between parent and adolescent.

Discuss the child's pubertal development and encourage the parents to discuss and consult with the pediatrician.

Promote independence and acceptance of responsibility. Assign chores around the house.

Encourage the adolescent to invite peers home.

Avoid denigrating the child's friends.

Problems and Plans

List here other issues and plans to address each of them, eg, acne, curfews, school performance.

Closing the Visit

♦ **Have your goals for this visit been met?**

♦ **Are there any other issues you want to discuss? This question should be asked of both the parent and the adolescent. Dealing with new concerns raised at this point may require a visit sooner than the next routine visit.**

♦ **Set up a time for the next visit.**

♦ **Indicate your availability should any concerns come up prior to the next scheduled visit. Encourage the adolescent to phone you as an important concern arises. Arrange with the adolescent and parent that the adolescent may schedule visits as necessary and that the parent will facilitate the visit (ie, transportation, fee payment), even if the adolescent does not want to share information about the visit with the parents. Reaffirm your guarantee of privacy.**

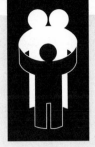

Health Supervision: 14- and 15-Year-Old Visit

Health Assessment

For many adolescents, this age represents the transition to middle adolescence. Puberty is well under way, even complete in many individuals. Preoccupations with the body and with attractiveness may decrease. At the same time, the lure and importance of the peer group increase and intensify. The peer group sets the standards for dress, recreation, behavior, and values. Many adolescents experiment with risk-taking behaviors. Conflicts with parents over issues of independence are at their highest peak at this time. Sexual exploration and experimentation are common. Recognition of sexual orientation occurs for many individuals in middle adolescence; for gay and lesbian youth such recognition may precipitate severe depression.

Interview With Behavioral Observations

Interviewing and examining adolescents privately, without parents present, acknowledges the adolescent's growing autonomy. Parents and caregivers may also desire the opportunity to provide information or to receive physician counseling without the adolescent present. However, entirely separate visits can create suspicion and distrust between the adolescent and parents. To meet the needs of both adolescents and their parents, physicians may bring the parents and adolescent together either for the welcoming portions or for the formulation. The remaining components of the visit can be conducted with each party individually.

The health care professional should explicitly discuss the rules of confidentiality with both adolescent and parents early in the interview. The adolescent's confidentiality should be respected unless information is revealed that indicates that the adolescent or another person is at serious risk. Health care professionals can alert the adolescent, prior to any discussion, that they will encourage the adolescent to discuss any problems with their parents, although the final decision about the content and timing of communication with the parents is the adolescent's.

Many experts favor the use of a previsit questionnaire (such as the Parent and Child Guides to Pediatric Visits included in Appendix C) to identify areas of concern, problems, and questions the adolescent may be encountering. Questions about eating, elimination, and sleep may be openers for some adolescents who are very private or reticent about talking. Priority should go to the issues of emotional well-being, school, friends, peer influences, and risk-taking behaviors such as sexual activity and use of alcohol and other drugs.

Welcoming questions (for the adolescent and parents)

How are things going for each of you?

To the adolescent: Are there particular issues or concerns you want to discuss at this visit?

To the parent: Are there particular issues or concerns you want to discuss at this visit?

Check on the status of issues addressed at the previous visit.

Establish the procedures for the remainder of the visit.

Specific questions for the adolescent

◆ **Nutrition**
What is your usual daily diet? What do you eat for breakfast? What do you eat for snacks? What do you think about your weight? What methods of dieting have you tried? How successful were you? Have you ever experienced binge eating?

◆ **Elimination**
Do you have any problems or concerns about urinating or having bowel movements? Do you have constipation or diarrhea? Have you experienced pain when urinating or wetting the bed during sleep?

◆ *For girls:* **Menstrual history**
When did you begin menstruating? How often does it occur? How long does it last? Have you experienced any bleeding between periods or any discharge, pain, or discomfort? Do you have any questions?

◆ **Sleep patterns**

How much sleep do you get on an average school night? On weekends?

◆ **School**

How's school going? How are your grades? What do you think about your grades? What do your parents say about your grades? What school activities or sports do you participate in? Any clubs? Have you thought about what you want to do when you grow up?

How many days did you miss from school this year? How many were excused absences and how many unexcused absences? Have you ever been in trouble at school? What were the circumstances?

◆ **Typical day**

What is a typical day like for you? How much television do you watch? How often do you play video games? Do you work? If so, how many hours? What responsibilities or chores do you have at home? Do you have any hobbies?

◆ **Social relationships/peer group influences**

Tell me about your friends. Who is your best friend? How often do you get together with friends? What do you and your friends like to do together? How easy is it for you to make new friends?

How are things going for you at home? How are family rules made and changed? What rules are you expected to follow? Do you think they are fair? How do your parents enforce the rules? What do you think about their methods? How are relationships with your siblings? Your parents? How is communication in the family? How could communication be improved? How does your family handle disagreements? Who do you confide in about your worries, concerns, and feelings? Do you feel you can talk to your parents about such issues?

◆ **Emotional well-being**

How would you describe yourself? What are you good at? What are you proud of? What makes you happy? What makes you sad? How much of the time do you feel sad?

What makes you angry? How do you express your anger in general? To your parents? How much of the time are you angry? Have you ever been so sad or angry that you thought about running away? Have you ever thought about hurting or killing yourself? Have you ever thought about hurting or killing someone else?

Have there been any changes or stresses in your family recently? What concerns do you have about your parents or siblings?

◆ **Health habits and risk assessment**

How do you rate your health? Your physical development? Your physical fitness? What questions or concerns do you have about changes in your body?

Many teens these days have tried smoking cigarettes. Does anyone you know smoke? Do any of your friends? How about you? How many cigarettes? How often?

Many teens these days have tried drinking. Does anyone you know drink? Among your friends does anyone drink? How about you? Have you ever been riding in a car with a driver who has been drinking? What did you do?

Many teens these days have tried marijuana or other illicit drugs. Has anyone you know? In your group of friends? How about you?

Many adolescents have developed a relationship with one "special" person. Have your friends paired up? How about you? Have you been attracted to members of the opposite sex? Same sex? Have you had sex with anyone? How often? What do you do to prevent sexually transmitted diseases? What do you do to prevent pregnancy? What is your strategy for avoiding HIV infection?

Many teens have experienced violence. Have any of your friends experienced violence? What are your experiences with violence? Have you ever been in trouble with the law?

Specific questions for the parent

How are things going for the family? How do you feel about being the parent of an adolescent? Do you have questions or concerns that you did not discuss when your child was present? Do you have any concerns about any of the following issues:

- ◆ grades
- ◆ school achievement
- ◆ absenteeism and truancy
- ◆ disobedience, aggressiveness, or antisocial behavior
- ◆ use of alcohol or other drugs
- ◆ depression, poor self-esteem, anxiety
- ◆ anorexia or bulimia
- ◆ lack of friends
- ◆ excessive peer influences
- ◆ sexual behavior or orientation

Have there been any changes in the family or household constellation? Have there been any recent stresses, illnesses, or crises since the last visit? Do you have special concerns about other family members (particularly about their abuse of alcohol or other drugs)?

Physical Examination With Behavioral Observations

The physical examination is usually completed without the parent present. It may be advisable for a nurse or chaperone to be with the physician and adolescent patient during the examination.

Measurements: *measure and plot percentiles*

- ◆ Height
- ◆ Weight
- ◆ Blood pressure

General physical examination

As part of the complete physical examination, make sure to include an evaluation of the Tanner stage. *The absence of a breast bud or of testicular enlargement by age 14 is evidence of delayed puberty and requires evaluation.* Note normal signs of gynecomastia in boys and asymmetrical breast development in girls. Screen adolescents for scoliosis with an upright forward bending test. Check for kyphosis. Evaluate the musculoskeletal system as a function of the adolescent's participation in sports and physical activity. Perform pelvic examinations for girls who are sexually active. Teach self-examination of the breasts or testes. Evaluate the skin for acne. Assess or reassess athletic girls and girls planning active involvement in sports for disordered eating, menstrual dysfunction, and decreased bone mineral density. Assess or reassess athletic boys and boys planning active involvement in sports for disordered eating. Perform objective assessments of vision and hearing unless performed at school and the results are normal and verifiable. Perform a pelvic examination on girls and conduct screening for sexually transmitted diseases as indicated.

Behavioral observations

Be concerned if the adolescent is timid, withdrawn, excessively fearful, or irritable.

Screening Procedures

A hematocrit or hemoglobin determination in menstruating females should be done annually, and urine dipstick analysis for leukocytes should be done at least once between 11 and 21 years of age but annually for sexually active children and adolescents. Perform cholesterol and hyperlipidemia screening if indicated by family history or risk factors such as smoking, hypertension, obesity, or diabetes mellitus are present. Perform a tuberculin skin test (Mantoux) if indicated (see Appendix F, Recommendations for Tuberculosis Testing).

A Papanicolaou (Pap) smear should be obtained annually for sexually active females. Adolescents who have had condyloma or abnormal Pap smears require more frequent screening. Sexually active females require annual gonorrhea and chlamydia screening.

Perform syphilis screening if the patient is sexually active or if requested by the patient. Perform human immunodeficiency virus (HIV) testing for adolescents who request the test and assenting adolescents who have any of the following risk factors:

- history of sexually transmitted diseases
- more than one sexual partner in the last 6 months
- intravenous drug use
- sexual intercourse with a partner at risk
- sex in exchange for drugs or money
- for males, sex with other males
- homelessness
- living in an endemic region

Formulation and Plan

Strengths of the Adolescent and Family

Describe some of the positive attributes of the child and family (eg, academic achievement, number of friends, or degree of self-reflection or self-control).

Health Maintenance

Immunizations

Check the adolescent's immunization status. Administer the second dose of the measles, mumps, and rubella (MMR) vaccine if not previously given. The vaccine should not be administered to pregnant females, and pregnancy must be avoided for 3 months after rubella administration. The hepatitis B series should be administered if not yet done. A tetanus-diphtheria (Td) booster should be administered every 10 years (see the current Recommended Childhood Immunization Schedule). Hepatitis A vaccine may be required in certain states or regions and for certain high-risk groups; consult your local public health authority.

Make sure to use and document the use of appropriate Vaccine Information Statements.*

Anticipatory guidance

Prioritize the issues discussed in the initial interview.

◆ **Nutrition**
Advise the adolescent directly about good health habits, including eating a well-balanced diet and avoiding junk food, excess salt and fat. It is important to eat breakfast daily. Weight can be maintained through a combination of sensible dietary intake and regular physical activity without the need for crash dieting, laxatives, or medication. Be alert to eating disorders and refer adolescents with these disorders for further assessment.

◆ **Sleep patterns**
Adolescents have erratic sleep patterns, but need on the average about 8 hours of sleep per night. They often deprive themselves of sleep during the week and catch up on weekends. Be alert to chronic sleep deprivation. Excessive sleeping or difficulties falling and staying asleep may indicate vegetative signs of depression.

◆ **Social development**
Discuss the issues of peer identification and resistance to peer pressure. Bring up specifics that include issues discussed at the beginning of the interview. Encourage age-appropriate peer activities and community service involvements. Suggest methods of resisting harmful peer pressure.

◆ **General health**
Discuss the wisdom of abstaining from smoking and using alcohol and other drugs.

*Vaccine Information Statements can be obtained from the AAP.

◆ **Injury prevention**

Anticipatory guidance about injury prevention should be tailored to the activities and risk factors of the individual. Middle adolescence is a period of high risk-taking behavior. The health professional must offer anticipatory guidance that is acceptable and motivating to the adolescent. Simple admonitions about what the adolescent should and should not do may be useless.

In communities in which violence and homicide are prevalent, personal safety and either potential or actual participation in violence should be discussed seriously with the adolescent.

Guns in the home are a danger to the family. If a gun is kept in the home, advise parents to store the gun and ammunition in locked, separate locations. (Pediatricians and other child health care professionals are urged to inform parents about the dangers of guns in and outside the home. The AAP recommends that pediatricians incorporate questions about guns into their patient history taking and urge parents who possess guns to remove them, especially handguns, from the home.)

For adolescents who are very active in sports, injury prevention should include warnings about overuse of muscles, fatigue, and specific stresses. Emphasize the importance of protective gear such as helmets and mouth guards. Reinforce the need for protective eyewear during participation in sports in which eye injury is a risk.

Many adolescents stop using the injury prevention measures that they used throughout childhood. They should be reminded to continue to wear bicycle helmets and to use seat belts. They should never get into a car with a stranger. They should be urged not to ride in cars when the driver has been drinking, using drugs, or acting recklessly. The responsibility involved with driving should be emphasized. Discuss the danger of riding unrestrained in the back of a pickup truck. Children younger than 16 years should not drive or ride on all-terrain vehicles.

The risks of alcohol and other drug abuse should be discussed. Illicit drugs introduce health risks because of uncertainty about their concentration or composition. In addition, abuse of alcohol and other drugs interferes with a person's insight, judgment, and self-control. Driving accidents and drowning frequently occur in individuals who are drunk. Sexual exploitation also occurs when individuals are under the influence of alcohol and other drugs.

At this age, adolescents can be advised to learn CPR for themselves, and issues of appropriate access to emergency medical systems can be discussed directly with the adolescent.

Reinforce the need for UV protection with the adolescent and parent.

◆ **Sexual activity**

Emphasize the advantages of abstinence.

If the adolescent is having sexual intercourse, discuss his or her feelings about it. Determine whether the adolescent draws a connection between sexual activity and intimacy and affection. Emphasize that it is appropriate to refuse sexual advances, particularly if they are unwelcome or forced, even if the individual has been sexually active previously. Encourage teens to report sexual abuse. Assist adolescents who want to avoid or discontinue sexual activity in planning for and practicing their approach to pressure.

For those who are sexually active or plan to become sexually active, stress mechanisms for preventing pregnancy and sexually transmitted diseases. Discuss how and where to buy latex condoms. Discuss strategies for avoiding HIV infection and acquired immunodeficiency syndrome (AIDS).

For all adolescents, see recommendations 16 through 19 of the American Medical Association "Guidelines for Preventive Services."*

◆ **Good parenting practices**

Suggest that parents include adolescents in establishing and enforcing fair rules for the home. Discipline of the adolescent serves as an educational tool, the same as in younger ages. For that reason, disciplinary action needs to catch the adolescent's attention and signal the severity of the rule infraction. The punishment should fit the offense. Many parents find that forbidding the adolescent to attend recreational activities (grounding) is an effective form of discipline.

Prepare parents for ambivalent feelings about their adolescent's increasing sexuality, emotions, and needs for independence from the family. Promoting independence and acceptance of responsibility demonstrates respect for and confidence in the adolescent.

Suggest that parents make every effort to maintain open and comfortable communication with the adolescent. This type of communication is fostered by attending events in which the adolescent is a participant and offering praise for the adolescent's school and extracurricular achievements. Open communication is also facilitated by the parents appreciating the adolescent's contributions at home, such as helping with chores. Despite these efforts, estrangement between parents and their adolescent is quite common.

Discuss the issues of the adolescent's privacy. Discourage violations of privacy (eg, bedroom, bathroom, mail, and phone calls). Adolescents should

---

*Elster AB, Kuznets NJ. *Guidelines for Adolescent Preventive Services.* Baltimore, MD: Williams & Wilkins; 1994.

be encouraged to make age-appropriate decisions and selections, including friends and activities.

Remind parents to continue to take their parental roles seriously. Parents serve as role models for behavior and moral judgment and in some circumstances may need to supervise potentially hazardous activities such as water sports or the use of power tools.

Encourage parents who are struggling with raising adolescent children to share their experiences with friends and families and to receive guidance, advice, and support from their pediatrician or other professional.

Problems and Plans

List issues and plans to address each of them (eg, if the adolescent has acne, plan a regimen of hygiene and prescribe medication; chronic cough, plan treatment to encourage smoking cessation).

Closing the Visit

◆ **Summarize major issues discussed during the visit.**

◆ **Have your goals for this visit been met?**

◆ **Are there any issues we missed? Ask questions to the adolescent and parent individually. New concerns raised late in the visit may require an additional scheduled visit before the next routine health maintenance visit.**

◆ **Set a time for the next appointment.**

◆ **Stress to the adolescent and to the parent your availability to deal with psychosocial, developmental, and school problems. Give the adolescent your card and invite him or her to call if issues arise. Obtain parental agreement for the adolescent to call or initiate a visit.**

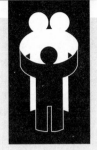

Health Supervision: 16- and 17-Year-Old Visit

Health Assessment

Most adolescents this age are in middle adolescence, although some are entering late adolescence. Puberty may be complete, particularly in girls. Preoccupations with the body and with attractiveness decrease after puberty. At the same time, the importance of the peer group may increase. The peer group sets the standards for dress, recreation, behavior, and values. Adolescents experiment with many risk-taking behaviors. Conflicts with parents over issues of independence are at their highest peak at this time. It is also a time of sexual exploration and experimentation. Recognition of sexual orientation occurs for many individuals in middle adolescence; for gay and lesbian youth such recognition may precipitate severe depression. At this stage the adolescent is frequently idealistic and altruistic. Plans for the future in terms of a career or relationship may still be rudimentary.

Interview With Behavioral Observations

At this age, a significant portion of the visit should take place without the parents present to acknowledge the adolescent's autonomy. The adolescent's confidentiality should be respected unless information is revealed that indicates that the adolescent or another person is at serious risk. Health care professionals can comment prior to any discussion that they will encourage the adolescent to discuss any problems with their parents, although the final decision about the content and timing of communication with the parents is the adolescent's.

An option remains to bring the adolescent, parent, and physician together for the initial portion of the session, discussing the chief concerns and goals for the visit and rules of confidentiality. The group can also be reunited for the summary. A previsit questionnaire remains an efficient method for surveying areas of questions or concerns (see Appendix C, Parent and Child Guides to Pediatric Visits).

Welcoming questions

How have things been going? How can I be helpful to you today?

Check on the status of issues addressed at the previous visit.

Obtain an interval history regarding the adolescent's health and well-being and the family circumstances.

Establish the procedures for the remainder of the visit.

Specific questions for the adolescent

◆ **Nutrition**

How is your diet? How many times a day do you eat? How satisfied are you with your weight and appearance? Have you ever used laxatives, medications, or forced yourself to throw up to lose weight? Have you ever been on a diet?

◆ **Elimination**

Do you have any problems or concerns about urination or your bowel movements?

◆ *For girls:* **Menstrual history**

When did you start menstruating? How often does it occur? How long does it last? Do you experience any bleeding between periods or any discharge, pain, or discomfort? Do you have any questions?

◆ **Sleep patterns**

How much sleep do you get on an average school night? On weekends? Do you have any trouble falling asleep, staying asleep, or waking up in the morning?

◆ **School**

How is school going? What were your grades on the last report card? How satisfied are you with your grades? How much pressure do you feel regarding grades? What are your plans for your future education? What do you need to accomplish to meet your goals? Have you thought about what you want to do when you grow up? How many days did you miss from school this year? Are your parents aware of your school absences? What were the reasons for the absences?

Have you ever been in trouble at school? What were the circumstances? Have you ever been in trouble with the law?

◆ **Typical day**

Have you started driving a car? What are your plans for learning how to drive? What rules have your parents established about your use of the car? What have you done to ensure the safety of your passengers?

Do you participate in any after-school activities, sports, or clubs? Do you have any hobbies? How much television do you watch? Do you play video games? Do you work? How many hours? Are there health risks at your job? What responsibilities or chores do you have at home?

◆ **Social relationships**

How is your relationship with your parents? How are things going for you at home? How are relationships with your siblings? Who do you confide in about your worries, concerns, and feelings? Can you discuss major problems or issues with your parents? How often do you experience conflict in your family? What causes the conflict? How are conflicts resolved?

Tell me about your friends. How often do you get together with friends? What do you and your friends like to do together? What do you think about these friendships?

Have you developed a steady relationship with someone? Have you been attracted to members of the opposite sex? The same sex? Have you had sex with anyone? How often? How will you decide when to have sexual relations? What do (will) you do to prevent sexually transmitted diseases? What do (will) you do to prevent pregnancy? What precautions do (will) you take to prevent human immunodeficiency virus (HIV) infection?

◆ **Emotional well-being**

How would you describe yourself? What are you good at? Proud of? What makes you happy? How often do you feel sad or angry? How have your feelings of sadness or anger affected your relationships, your school performance, and your sense of well-being? Have you ever considered yourself depressed?

◆ **Risk-taking behavior**

What education have you received about tobacco and smoking? What did you think about it? Do you smoke or chew tobacco? How often?

Do you drink alcoholic beverages? What types? How often? How much? Have you ever been riding in a car with a driver who has been drinking? What did you do? Have you ever been pressured to do things while under the influence of alcohol?

Are you worried about any of your friends using marijuana or other drugs? Have you ever used them? How often? What was the effect on you?

Have you ever been in trouble with the law? What were the circumstances?

Questions about the family

Have there been any changes in the family or household constellation? Have there been any recent stresses, illnesses, or crises since the last visit? Do you have special concerns about other family members, particularly concerning abuse of alcohol or other drugs?

For the parent: How are things going for the family? How do you feel about being the parent of an adolescent? Do you have questions or concerns that you did not discuss when your child was present?

What do you think about your adolescent's school performance, activities, and friendships? Do you have any concerns about your child's behaviors, safety, or well-being? Have you addressed these concerns with your child?

Physical Examination With Behavioral Observations

The physical examination is usually completed without the parent present. It is advisable for a nurse or chaperone to be with the physician and adolescent patient during the examination.

Measurements: *measure and plot percentiles*

- ◆ Height
- ◆ Weight
- ◆ Blood pressure

General physical examination

As part of the complete physical examination, make sure to include an evaluation of the Tanner stage. The absence of a breast bud or of testicular enlargement is evidence of delayed puberty and requires evaluation. Note gynecomastia in boys and asymmetrical breast development in girls. Assess or reassess athletic girls and girls planning active involvement in sports for disordered eating, menstrual dysfunction, and decreased bone mineral density. Assess or reassess athletic boys and boys planning active involvement in sports for disordered eating.

Screen the adolescent who has not completed growing for scoliosis with a forward bending test. Check for kyphosis. Evaluate the musculoskeletal system as a function of the adolescent's participation in sports and physical activity. Perform a pelvic examination for adolescent girls who are sexually active. Teach the adolescent self-examination of the breasts or testicles. Examine the skin for acne.

Perform subjective assessments of vision and hearing.

Observations of behavior and development

Be concerned if the adolescent is withdrawn or irritable.

Screening Procedures

A hematocrit or hemoglobin determination should be done on menstruating adolescents annually. A dipstick urinalysis for leukocytes should be done for males and females at least once between the ages of 11 and 21 but annually for sexually active children and adolescents.

Perform cholesterol screening if indicated (see the 2-year-old visit) or if a family history is unavailable and risk factors such as smoking, hypertension, obesity, or diabetes mellitus are present.

A Papanicolaou (Pap) smear should be obtained for sexually active females. Adolescents who have had condyloma or abnormal Pap smears require more frequent screening. Sexually active females require annual gonorrhea and chlamydia screening.

Screen for sexually transmitted diseases if patient is sexually active. Perform HIV testing for adolescents who request it and encourage testing for any of the following risk factors:

- ◆ History of sexually transmitted diseases
- ◆ More than one sexual partner in the last 6 months
- ◆ Intravenous drug use
- ◆ Sexual intercourse with a partner at risk
- ◆ Sex in exchange for drugs or money
- ◆ For males: sex with other males
- ◆ Homelessness

In addition, HIV testing should be considered for individuals who received blood transfusions prior to 1985.

Perform a tuberculin skin test (Mantoux) if indicated for high-risk factors (see Appendix F, Recommendations for Tuberculosis Testing).

Formulation and Plan

Strengths of the Child and Family

Describe some of the positive attributes of the adolescent and family (eg, academic achievement, peer group activities, degree of self-reflection or self-control). Acknowledge the positive aspects of the parent-adolescent relationship.

Health Maintenance

Immunizations

Check the adolescent's immunization status. Administer the second dose of measles, mumps, and rubella (MMR) vaccine if not previously given. The vaccine must not be administered to pregnant females, and pregnancy must be avoided for 3 months after administration. A hepatitis B series should be administered if not previously given. A tetanus-diphtheria (Td) booster needs to be administered every 10 years (see the current Recommended Childhood Immunization Schedule). Hepatitis A vaccine may be required in certain states or regions and for certain high-risk groups; consult your local public health authority.

Document the use of the appropriate Vaccine Information Statements.*

Anticipatory guidance

◆ Nutrition

Recognize that many adolescents may be purchasing or preparing a lot of the food they eat. Advise the adolescent about good health habits including eating a well-balanced diet and avoiding junk food and excess salt and fat. Provide counseling and/or a referral to adolescents who resort to crash dieting, laxatives, medications, or forced emesis for weight control.

◆ Sleep patterns

Remind the adolescent that on the average adolescents require about 8 hours of sleep per night. Adolescents have erratic sleep patterns, often depriving themselves of sleep during the week and catching up on the weekends. Be alert to chronic sleep deprivation. Excessive sleeping or difficulties falling and staying asleep may constitute vegetative signs of depression.

◆ Social relationships

Encourage peer group activities and community involvement. Discuss the issues of peer identification and the need for adolescents to resist some peer pressure. Suggest and practice specific methods of resisting peer pressure.

◆ Injury prevention

Anticipatory guidance about injury prevention should be tailored to the activities and risk factors of the individual. Middle adolescence is a period of high risk-taking behavior. The health professional must offer anticipatory guidance that is acceptable and motivating to the adolescent. Simple admonitions about what the adolescent should do and not do may be useless.

---

*Vaccine Information Statements can be obtained from the AAP.

Review driving safety for adolescents who have begun driving or are planning to learn to drive. Stress the responsibility of driving a car. Although 16- and 17-year-olds are old enough to operate all-terrain vehicles (ATVs), they should understand that ATVs must not be operated on the road. Review safe operation of personal watercraft. Discuss safety issues while operating or riding as a passenger on snowmobiles.

Remind the adolescent to use seat belts and to insist that passengers in the car use seat belts. Urge the adolescent not to get into a car with a driver who has been drinking, using drugs, or acting reckless. Remind the adolescent that driving accidents and drowning frequently occur in individuals who are drunk.

The risks of alcohol and other drug abuse should be discussed. Illicit drugs introduce health risks because of the uncertainty about their concentration or composition. In addition, abuse of alcohol and other drugs interferes with a person's insight, judgment, and self-control. Sexual exploitation also occurs when individuals are under the influence of alcohol and other drugs.

For adolescents who use alcohol or other drugs, differentiate among experimentation, regular use, dependence, and abuse. Discourage experimentation. Make appropriate referrals for regular use, dependence, and abuse.

For adolescents who smoke or use tobacco products, encourage participation in a smoking cessation program and discuss other smoking cessation strategies.

In communities in which violence and homicide are prevalent, the adolescent's safety and participation in violence should be discussed. Participation in violent behavior often occurs when the individual is under the influence of alcohol or other drugs.

Guns in the home are a danger to the family. If a gun is kept in the home, advise parents to keep the gun and ammunition in locked, separate locations. (Pediatricians and other child health care professionals are urged to inform parents about the dangers of guns in and outside the home. The AAP recommends that pediatricians incorporate questions about guns into their patient history taking and urge parents who possess guns to remove them, especially handguns, from the home.)

For adolescents who are very active in sports, injury prevention should include wearing proper equipment, avoiding overexercising, fatigue, and specific stresses. Reinforce the need for protective eyewear during participation in sports with a risk of eye injury.

Reinforce the need for UV protection with the adolescent and parent.

Reinforce the need for smoke detectors in the home.

◆ **Sexual activity**

Encourage abstinence.

If the adolescent is having sexual intercourse, discuss his or her feelings about it. Emphasize that it is appropriate to refuse unwanted or forced sexual advances and to report sexual abuse. Assist adolescents who want to avoid or discontinue sexual activity in planning for and practicing their approach to pressure.

For those who are sexually active or plan to become sexually active, stress mechanisms for preventing pregnancy and sexually transmitted diseases. Discuss how to buy and wear condoms. Discuss AIDS.

◆ **Good parenting practices**

Suggest that parents include adolescents in establishing and enforcing fair rules for the home. Discuss the parents' attitudes toward driving. Assist the parents in establishing fair rules for use of the car. The punishments should fit the offense. Grounding or prohibiting phone calls may be effective forms of discipline.

Prepare parents for ambivalent feelings about their adolescent's sexuality and increasing needs for independence from the family. Promoting independence and acceptance of responsibility demonstrates respect for and confidence in the adolescent.

Suggest that parents make every effort to maintain open, comfortable communication with the adolescent. This type of communication is fostered by attending events in which the adolescent is a participant and offering praise for the adolescent's school and extracurricular achievements. Open communication is also facilitated by the parents' appreciating the adolescent's contributions at home, such as helping with chores. Despite these efforts, estrangement between parents and the adolescent is quite common.

Discuss the issues of the adolescent's privacy. Discourage violations of privacy (eg, bedroom, bathroom, mail, and telephone calls). Adolescents should be encouraged to make age-appropriate decisions and selections, including friends and activities. Denigrating an adolescent's friends may precipitate problems in the parent-adolescent relationship or compromise self-esteem.

Encourage parents who are struggling with raising adolescent children to share their experiences with friends and families to receive guidance, advice, and support from their pediatrician or other professional.

Problems and Plans

List problems identified and plan for managing each one (eg, "Mom doesn't want me only hanging out during this summer," assist in investigating volunteer or salaried position; if the examination reveals visible dental caries, discuss the need for increased attention to oral hygiene and recommend that the adolescent schedule a visit with the dentist).

Closing the Visit

♦ **Acknowledge the positive aspects of the parent-adolescent relationship.**

♦ **Make sure that expectations and needs have been met.**

♦ **Ask the child and parent individually: Are there any issues we missed? New concerns raised late in the visit may require an additional scheduled visit before the next routine health maintenance visit.**

♦ **Stress to the adolescent your availability. Mention interest in and willingness to aid in the assessment or treatment of psychosocial, developmental, and school problems. Provide specific circumstances that should warrant a return, such as decline in school performance, withdrawal from friends and family, signs of depression, or related issues. Give the adolescent your card and invite him or her to call if issues arise. Obtain parental agreement for the adolescent to call or initiate a visit.**

♦ **Set a time for the next appointment.**

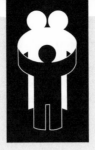

Health Supervision: 18- and 19-Year-Old Visit

Health Assessment

In late adolescence, emancipation is nearly complete, and there is increased interest in career choice. Social skills become enhanced, and long-term, intimate physical and psychological relationships develop. Body image and gender role definition are nearly completed.

Interview With Behavioral Observations

Behavioral observations are made during both the interview and the physical examination. Parental presence is rarely required for the visit since the late adolescent should be able to provide history and understand anticipatory counseling. The previsit questionnaire is an efficient method for systematically obtaining historical and psychosocial information (see Appendix C, Parent and Child Guides to Pediatric Visits).

Assess the adolescent-physician interaction. Consider whether the adolescent is friendly, cooperative, verbal, and trusting. Of concern is the late adolescent who is tense, shy, guarded, hostile, or provocative.

Welcoming questions

How have you been since I saw you last? How are things going? What should we discuss at the visit today?

The major concerns of the late adolescent may include future plans for college, a career, marriage, and peer relations. Common problems at this age include pressure to engage in sexual relations, somatic complaints, loneliness, discouragement, eating disorders, suicidal thoughts, menstrual disorders, use of alcohol or other drugs, acne, and anxiety.

Check on the status of issues addressed at the previous visit.

Since I saw you last, have you had any illnesses, hospitalizations, allergies, trauma, immunizations, major changes at home (illness, death, unemployment, separation, divorce, remarriage, relocation of household members)?

Specific questions about the adolescent

◆ **Nutrition**

How have you been eating? Do you eat a balanced diet? Do you take any supplements, such as iron or vitamins? What is your assessment of your weight and personal appearance? What methods do you use to lose or gain weight? Do you receive routine dental care? Do you floss regularly?

◆ **Elimination**

Do you have concerns about the frequency and consistency of your bowel movements? Do you experience any discomfort? Do you experience urgency? Dysuria? Nocturia? Wetting?

◆ *For women:* **Menstrual history**

How frequently do you menstruate? How long are your periods? When was your last menstrual period? How much discomfort do you experience? Do you take any medications to relieve cramping or pain? Any vaginal discharge?

◆ **School or work**

What are you doing these days? How is your education proceeding? Are you satisfied with your progress? What are your future plans?

How is your job going? How is your salary? How are the work conditions? What are your long-term goals?

◆ **Social relationships**

Whom do you confide in about your worries, concerns, or feelings? How is your relationship with your family? Are you worried about the health of any family member?

Tell me about your friends. Do you confide in your friends? What do you do when you're with your friends? Have you thought about what all the freedom will be like when you are working full-time? Will you live at home or move out? How do you think you'll manage it?

Are you attracted to members of the opposite sex? Same sex? Do you date? Are you going steady? Is the relationship emotionally or physically intimate? Are you sexually active? If so, are there any problems with your sexual activity you'd like to discuss? Are you involved in any violent relationships at home or with other people your age?

◆ **Emotional well-being**

What do you do for fun? Do you participate in sports or have a hobby? What do you think about your level of fitness?

What do you do the best? Enjoy the most? What do you have to do that you don't enjoy or do poorly? What two or three things would you like to do even better? What kind of changes would you like to see in yourself? How do you think your personal thoughts differ from those of other adolescents? Your values? Interests? Feelings? Hopes? Do you practice any religion? What makes you angry? What do you do when you get angry? Would you say you are generally happy?

◆ **Health habits and risk assessment**

Do you smoke? How many cigarettes do you smoke daily? Do you want to stop? Why not?

Do you drink? How much? How often? When was the last time you were drunk? What happened when you were drunk? Do you ever drive or ride in a car with someone driving who has been drinking alcohol or using other drugs?

Do you use alcohol or other drugs? What kind? How often? How do you feel about your drug use? Are you involved in any violent relationships at home or with people your age? Have you gotten in trouble with the law? Are you involved in any sexual activity against your will?

Physical Examination With Behavioral Observations

Measurements: *measure and plot percentiles*

◆ Height

◆ Weight

◆ Blood pressure

General physical examination

As part of the complete physical examination, make sure to include an evaluation of the Tanner stage, vision screening, hearing screening, an evaluation of sports fitness, and a pelvic examination if the adolescent is sexually active or has menstrual problems; instruct the adolescent in self-examination of breasts or testicles. Assess or reassess athletic girls and girls planning active involvement in sports for disordered eating, menstrual dysfunction, and decreased bone mineral density. Assess or reassess athletic boys and boys planning active involvement in sports for disordered eating. It may be appropriate to have a nurse or chaperone in the room during physical examination.

Observations of behavior and development

Be concerned if the adolescent is withdrawn or irritable.

Screening Procedures

A hematocrit or hemoglobin determination should be done on menstruating adolescents annually. A urine dipstick for leukocytes should be done on all teenagers once between 11 and 21 years but annually for sexually active adolescents.

Perform cholesterol screening (nonfasting) if indicated by a family history of elevated cholesterol levels or by the adolescent's risk factors (smoking, hypertension, obesity, diabetes mellitus, or excessive consumption of dietary saturated fats and cholesterol). A fasting lipoprotein analysis should be done if the adolescent's cholesterol level is elevated or if there is a family history of coronary artery disease, peripheral vascular disease, cerebrovascular disease, or sudden cardiac death at or before age 55.

A pelvic examination and a Papanicolaou smear should be offered between the ages of 18 and 21 years. Sexually active adolescents should be tested for syphilis, hepatitis B (if not fully immunized), gonorrhea, and chlamydia. Human immunodeficiency virus testing should be encouraged if the young adult is at risk (has multiple sexual partners, a history of two or more episodes of sexually transmitted disease, or high-risk homosexual behavior); males who have participated in homosexual behavior should also be screened for anal and oral gonorrhea. Perform a tuberculin (Mantoux) test if indicated (see Appendix F, Recommendations for Tuberculosis Testing).

Formulation and Plan

Strengths of the Adolescent

Reinforce the strengths of the adolescent with comments such as, "I'm very impressed that you are able to keep a job and go to vocational school at the same time," "I'm happy to hear that your group of friends is doing volunteer work at the senior citizen home," or "It's really good that you are committed to using birth control for now so you can finish school, even though so many of your friends are already having babies."

Health Maintenance

Immunizations

After the adolescent's 18th birthday, he or she can read the Vaccine Information Statements* and discuss the pros and cons of vaccination if they are given at this visit.

Make sure all immunizations are up-to-date, including the second dose of measles, mumps, and rubella (MMR) vaccine. Girls should not become pregnant for 3 months after vaccination.

Administer a tetanus-diphtheria (Td) booster every 10 years. Administer a hepatitis B series if not previously done (see the current Recommended Childhood Immunization Schedule). Hepatitis A vaccine may be required in certain states or regions and for certain high-risk groups; consult your local public health authority.

Anticipatory guidance

Much anticipatory guidance can be done during the interview as specific issues come up.

- ◆ **Nutrition**
  Review the value of a balanced diet and the danger of eating fads.

  Continue brushing teeth twice a day, flossing regularly, and having regular dental checkups.

- ◆ **General health habits**
  Review the importance of

  - ❖ Maintaining appropriate weight.
  - ❖ Regular physical activity.
  - ❖ Avoidance of anabolic steroids, cigarettes, smokeless tobacco, illicit drugs, and locations where tobacco smoke is present. (For adolescents who smoke or use tobacco products, encourage participation in a smoking cessation program and discuss other smoking cessation strategies.)
  - ❖ Sufficient amounts of sleep.

- ◆ **Injury prevention**
  Discuss the regular use of sunscreen to avoid sunburn.

  Adolescents should drive responsibly, never drive or ride in a car with a driver who has been drinking or using drugs, and never get into a car with a stranger. Discuss the danger of riding unrestrained in the back of a pickup truck. Seat belts should always be used.

---

*Vaccine Information Statements can be obtained from the AAP.

Discuss the importance of recognizing and avoiding situations of potential physical or sexual abuse.

Guns in the home are a danger to the family. If a gun is kept in the home, advise parents to store the gun and ammunition in locked, separate locations. (Pediatricians and other child health care professionals are urged to inform parents about the dangers of guns in and outside the home. The AAP recommends that pediatricians incorporate questions about guns into their patient history taking and urge parents who possess guns to remove them, especially handguns, from the home.)

Adolescents should be reminded of the dangers of violence. Review strategies to resolve interpersonal conflicts without violence.

Reinforce safety issues while operating or riding as a passenger on snowmobiles.

Reinforce the need for smoke detectors in the home.

◆ **Social relationships**

Discuss changing communication patterns within the family, with parents, siblings, and extended family members.

Discuss handling separation from home. Inform the adolescent of where medical services may be obtained when away from home (eg, college health center, community family planning clinic, or a community practitioner).

◆ **Sexual activity**

If the adolescent is sexually active, discuss his or her feelings about sex. If the adolescent is uneasy or fearful about being sexually active, offer support and specific suggestions for managing vulnerable situations. Emphasize that it is appropriate to say "no."

Caution against relationships involving physical violence or emotional abuse.

For those who plan to continue or initiate sexual activity, offer contraceptive advice and discuss methods of preventing sexually transmitted diseases. Provide information on acquired immunodeficiency syndrome and its prevention.

Remind the adolescent that the fewer the number of lifetime sexual partners, the lower the health risk.

◆ **Future plans**

Discuss earning money, chores, sports, hobbies, and studying.

Discuss college or vocational education, work or career, marriage, and child-rearing. Suggest discussing the career possibility with an acquaintance who is in that field to learn what it is like.

Problems and Plans

List specific problems and plans for their management.

Closing the Visit

◆ Have your goals been met?

◆ Is there anything else we should talk about?

◆ Issues raised at this time may require another appointment.

◆ Schedule the next visit. Remind the adolescent that you will provide his or her care until 21 years of age (or whatever the specifics of your practice are) and that annual checkups should continue.

◆ Advise the adolescent who is going away to college that the school will have a student health service to handle any problems, including contraception and venereal disease.

◆ Remind the adolescent that you are available if issues should come up before the next scheduled visit.

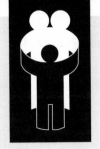

Health Supervision: 20- and 21-Year-Old Visit

Health Assessment

By this age, emancipation is completed for some late adolescents and in process for others. Career choice may be a major concern for some individuals. Social skills become enhanced and intimate physical and psychological relationships occur. Body image and gender role definition are generally completed. It is appropriate to plan for the transition to an adult health care professional.

Interview With Behavioral Observations

Parental presence is not usually required, although in rare situations it may be appropriate. A previsit questionnaire is a mechanism for identifying areas of concern, problems, or questions (see Appendix C, Parent and Child Guides to Pediatric Visits). Priority should go to the issues of emotional well-being, school or employment, intimate relationships, and risk-taking behaviors such as engaging in sexual activity and the use of alcohol or other drugs.

Welcoming questions

How are things going for you? What issues or concerns would you like to discuss at this visit?

Check on the status of issues addressed at the previous visit.

Specific questions to the adolescent

◆ Nutrition

What is your usual daily diet? How do you learn about nutrition? Tell me about your eating habits.

◆ Elimination

What are the frequency and consistency of your bowel movements? How frequently do you urinate? Do you experience dysuria or nocturia?

◆ *For women:* Menstrual history

How often do you menstruate? How long does your period last? Do you experience any bleeding between periods or any discharge or discomfort? What was the date of your last menstrual period?

◆ Sleep patterns

How much sleep do you get on an average school or work night? On weekends?

◆ School and work

How's school or work going? What do you think about your grades? Your boss? How many days did you miss from school or work this year? What are the reasons for missed school or work? What are your future plans?

◆ Social relationships

Tell me about your friends. How often do you get together with friends? Is it easy for you to make friends? Is there a special person in your life? Who? How long have you known each other? How intimate physically and emotionally is the relationship? Are you having sexual intercourse? How do you prevent pregnancy? Sexually transmitted diseases? What is your strategy for avoiding human immunodeficiency virus (HIV)? Whom do you confide in about your worries, concerns, feelings? How do or how would your parents handle such a discussion?

◆ Emotional well-being

How would you describe yourself? What are you good at? Proud of? What makes you happy? What makes you sad? How much of the time do you feel sad? Have you ever thought about hurting or killing yourself? What makes you angry? How do you express your anger in general? To your parents? How much of the time are you angry?

◆ Health habits and risk assessment

How do you rate your health? Your physical development? Your physical fitness?

Do you smoke cigarettes? How many daily? How do you feel about your smoking? What would it take to help you quit smoking?

Do you drink alcohol? What type of alcohol do you like? How much do you drink ordinarily? When was the last time you drank? How much did you drink then? How often do you get drunk? Do you ever drive after drinking alcohol? Do you ever ride in a car after the driver has been drinking? What impact has alcohol had on your life? How would you know if you needed to quit drinking? How would you approach quitting?

Do you use other drugs? What types? How much? How often? What impact have drugs had on your life?

◆ **Questions about the family or household**
With whom are you living? How are things at home? How is communication with your family? How could communication be improved? Have there been any changes in the family or household constellation? Have there been any recent stresses, illnesses, or crises since the last visit? Do you have special concerns about other family members (particularly about violent behavior or the abuse of alcohol or other drugs)?

Physical Examination With Behavioral Observations

The physical examination is completed in private. It may be advisable for a nurse or chaperone to be with the physician and adolescent patient during the examination.

Measurements: *measure and plot percentiles*

◆ Height

◆ Weight

◆ Blood pressure

General physical examination

As part of the complete physical examination, evaluate the musculoskeletal system as a function of the adolescent's participation in sports and physical activity. Perform pelvic examinations for adolescent girls who are sexually active. Teach the adolescent self-examination of the breasts or testicles. Observe behavior and development. Assess vision and hearing.

Screening Procedures

A hematocrit or hemoglobin determination should be done on menstruating adolescents annually. A urine dipstick for leukocytes should be done at least once between 11 and 21 years of age but annually for sexually active adolescents. Perform cholesterol screening if indicated by family history, if a family history is unavailable, and/or risk factors such as smoking, hypertension, obesity, or diabetes mellitus are present. A pelvic examination and a Papanicolaou (Pap) smear should be offered between the ages of 18 and 21 years. A Pap smear should be obtained for sexually active females. Adolescents who have had condyloma or abnormal Pap smears require more frequent screening. Sexually active females require annual gonorrhea and chlamydia screening. Asymptomatic sexually active males can be screened with a urine dipstick for leukocytes. Syphilis screening is needed for sexually active patients. Screening for HIV infection is necessary for adolescents who request the test or who have any of the following risk factors and consent to the test:

- History of sexually transmitted diseases
- More than one sexual partner in the last 6 months
- Intravenous drug use
- Sexual intercourse with a partner at risk
- Sex in exchange for drugs or money
- *For males:* sex with other males
- Homelessness

In addition, HIV testing should be considered for individuals who received blood transfusions prior to 1985. A tuberculin skin test (Mantoux) should be performed if indicated (see Appendix F, Recommendations for Tuberculosis Testing).

Formulation and Plan

Strengths of the Adolescent

Reinforce positive attributes of the patient's life that have been discussed during the visit. Comment on achievements in a job, school, community activity, or personal relationship when appropriate. Praise young adults for evidence of increasing independence.

Health Maintenance

Immunizations

Check the adolescent's immunization status. Administer the second dose of measles, mumps, and rubella (MMR) vaccine if not previously given. The vaccine must not be administered to pregnant females, and pregnancy must be avoided for 3 months after administration. A hepatitis B series should be administered if not previously given. A tetanus-diphtheria (Td) booster needs to be administered every 10 years (see the current Recommended Childhood Immunization Schedule).

Document the use of Vaccine Information Statements.*

Anticipatory guidance

Prioritize the issues discussed in the initial interview. Anticipatory guidance about injury prevention should be tailored to the activities and risk factors of the individual. The health professional must offer anticipatory guidance that is acceptable and motivating to the adolescent. Simple admonitions about what and what not to do may be useless.

◆ **Nutrition**
Advise the adolescent directly about good health habits, including eating a well-balanced diet and avoiding junk food and excess salt and fat. It is important to eat breakfast daily. Weight can be maintained through a combination of sensible dietary intake and regular physical activity without the need for crash dieting. Routine teeth brushing and regular dental care are also important.

◆ **Sleep patterns**
Remind the adolescent that, on the average, about 8 hours of sleep a day is necessary. Be alert to chronic sleep deprivation. Excessive sleeping or difficulties falling and staying asleep may constitute vegetative signs of depression.

◆ **Social relationships**
Discuss issues around establishing intimacy. Bring up specifics in terms of issues discussed during the data gathering.

◆ **Injury prevention**
In communities in which violence and homicide are prevalent, the adolescent's participation in violent activities and safety issues need to be seriously discussed.

For adolescents who are very active in sports, injury prevention should include warnings about overuse of muscles, fatigue, and specific stresses. Reinforce the need for protective eyewear during participation in sports with a risk of eye injury.

Many adolescents discontinue the injury prevention behaviors that they used throughout childhood. They should be reminded to continue to wear bicycle helmets and to use seat belts. They should be urged not to ride in a car when the driver has been drinking, using drugs, or acting recklessly.

---

*Vaccine Information Statements can be obtained from the AAP.

The risks of alcohol and other drugs should be discussed. Illicit drug use introduces health risks because of uncertainty about the concentration or composition of the drug. In addition, abuse of alcohol and other drugs interferes with a person's insight, judgment, and self-control. Driving accidents and drowning frequently occur when individuals are drunk. Sexual exploitation also occurs when individuals are under the influence of alcohol and other drugs.

For adolescents who smoke or use tobacco products, encourage participation in a smoking cessation program and discuss other smoking cessation strategies.

Reinforce the need for UV protection with the young adult.

Reinforce safety issues while operating or riding as a passenger on snowmobiles.

Reinforce the need for smoke detectors in the home.

◆ **Sexual activity**
If the adolescent is having sexual intercourse, discuss his or her feelings about it. Connect sexual activity with intimacy and affection. Emphasize that it is appropriate to refuse sexual advances, particularly if they are unwelcome or if the adolescent feels forced into it. Assist adolescents who want to avoid or discontinue sexual activity in planning for and practicing their approach to pressure.

For adolescents who are sexually active or plan to become sexually active, stress mechanisms for preventing pregnancy and preventing sexually transmitted diseases. Discuss how and where to buy condoms. Discuss acquired immunodeficiency syndrome.

Problems and Plans

Highlight issues and plans to address each of them (eg, for elevated cholesterol levels, review the adolescent's diet and exercise plan, repeat test in 1 year; for onset of wheezing, provide a medication regimen, discuss possible allergies, and advise the adolescent to stop smoking).

Closing the Visit

◆ Have your goals for this visit been met?

◆ Have any issues been missed? New concerns raised late in the visit may require an additional scheduled visit before the next routine health maintenance visit.

◆ Review your policy for age of patients. Set a time for the next appointment if the young adult will be seeing you. Review the transition of the adolescent to another health care professional if indicated. Provide written record of immunizations, tuberculin tests, and ongoing health concerns.

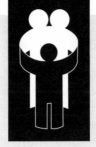

Clinical Approaches to Common Issues During Health Supervision

Introduction to Supplements

Guidelines for Health Supervision III recommends that each scheduled health supervision visit serve to assess multiple complex domains — physical health, immunization status, behavioral traits, developmental progress, family relationships, school performance, risks to health, and risk-taking behavior — that impinge significantly on the health and well-being of children. The interview becomes an open dialogue with the family and child, driven in large part by their issues, questions, and concerns. Observations of parent-child interactions and child reactions during physical examinations offer additional opportunities for gathering data and exchanging information. *Guidelines for Health Supervision III* encourages practitioners to conceptualize the scope of health supervision as broad and deep.

One of the major barriers for health professionals when they assume this intense strategy for comprehensive health supervision is their concern about how to proceed when a problem is identified. Practitioners must be familiar with the common concerns that arise in health supervision and with general approaches to the design of interventions. The supplements that follow meet two goals: first, to describe and categorize problems that arise frequently in the course of health supervision and second, to provide a general and theoretically sound framework that the health professional can apply to these problems.

The organization of the supplements follows the organization of data gathering, which is presented in the preceding chapters. One or two representative topics are included for each domain. "Feeding Behavior in Infancy and Early Childhood" addresses issues that arise in the discussion of feeding, eating, and nutrition. "Temper Tantrums" addresses causes of and solutions to these common occurrences. "Toilet Training" discusses this major accomplishment during the toddler years and describes common problems in achieving continence. "Sleep Problems" are discussed frequently. "Individual Differences" and "Effective Discipline" discuss temperamental and behavioral characteristics of individual children, and "Self-Comforting Behaviors" interprets thumb-sucking, masturbation, and other repetitive behaviors as strategies that children use to control their own emotional states and the environment around them. "Parental Stress and the Child at Risk" explores aspects of family functioning. Pediatricians are encouraged to learn more about these and other topics commonly encountered in health supervision.

These supplements provide health practitioners with general direction on selected topics. The absence of "cookbook" specificity is intentional; it follows from the model of health supervision that these guidelines promote. Health practitioners should avoid pat advice and simplistic prescriptions for complex problems. Practitioners must listen intently to the issues as they emerge in the context of a particular child, family, and community. The health supervision visit is an opportunity to explore the issues — the nature and course of the symptom, its meaning and impact within the family, the success or failure of previous attempts by the family or school or community to address the problem, and the current degree of motivation. Interventions are more effective when the child and family participate in their design and when they are tailored to the individual situation in a family centered and culturally sensitive approach.

The chapters that follow serve as a guide and a framework for anticipatory guidance and psychosocial interventions. Health practitioners are urged to integrate the information provided in the chapters with the specific circumstances of children and families in practicing health promotion, preventive care, and behavioral medicine.

Feeding Behavior in Infancy and Early Childhood

The development of feeding skills is a complex process, depending on the motor, emotional, and social maturation of the child as well as on the child's temperament and relationship with the family members. Many constitutional and environmental factors may help or hinder feeding progress. Frequently, parental concerns relate more to the child's eating style or the parents' unrealistic expectations about the amount of food consumption than to the child's nutritional state. The development of feeding skills is detailed in the Table, together with some common concerns occurring at each stage. The pattern of food consumption is dependent on the child's developmental skills. Clinical evaluation and counseling about feeding behavior is most effective in the context of developmental readiness.

Anticipatory Guidance

Many parents equate feeding their children with their success as caregivers. Children who do not fulfill parental expectations about food intake are often teased, urged, bribed, or made to feel guilty. Consequently, children learn that their actions at mealtime may attract attention or even precipitate some other family reaction. Eventually, the feeding situation may be used by some children as the opportunity to exercise control over the family. Thus, successful management of feeding problems begins by anticipating common developmental-psychosocial issues that surround feeding and enabling families to avoid or cope better with such issues should they arise.

During health supervision visits, parents should be informed about the normal development of feeding skills, about diet and caloric requirements at different ages, and about the variable appetites of individual children. Helping parents to recognize the child's readiness signs, such as reaching for a cup or increased interest in the environment while nursing, may lead to easy weaning from the breast or bottle. Parental anxiety can be avoided if parents are prepared for the usual decrease in appetite as the infant enters the toddler stage. In addition, realization that children do not need to eat a great variety of foods, but may get adequate nutrition through a limited selection of foods with good nutritional value (eg, fruit instead of vegetable) can be reassuring. Families that are fastidious may be reluctant to allow children to feed themselves because of the "mess" they create; these concerns should be addressed by focusing parental concern on the child's emerging autonomy and need to experiment — even at mealtime!

Pediatric Intervention

When the parents complain — or the pediatrician suspects — that a feeding problem exists, the following areas should be explored:

◆ What is the present mealtime experience?

◆ Is there consistency in mealtime routines?

◆ What is the child's feeding history?

◆ Has the child been allowed to explore and initiate activity in other areas?

◆ Has the child been able to achieve competence in other areas?

◆ Is the child's growth appropriate? Demonstration of the child's progress in weight and height on a growth chart is often reassuring.

◆ Are there any other areas of concern about the child's behavior?

◆ What is the child's general health state? Is the child perceived as vulnerable or in special need of being fed for some reason?

◆ What are the family's cultural and social values associated with food?

◆ Do parental attitudes contribute to the problem?

With this background knowledge to help individualize problem management, the following general guidelines for parents can be used to help with feeding:

◆ Encourage self-feeding when the child is developmentally capable, usually by 9 months. Use child-appropriate items such as two-handled plastic cups.

◆ Offer small portions with the opportunity for additional helpings.

◆ Offer a variety of healthful food items. Allow the child to choose from two or three foods at a time (especially important during period of developing autonomy).

◆ Offer praise liberally.

◆ Limit the length of meals to a predetermined maximum time. Allow the child to eat with rest of family at least some of the time.

◆ Be consistent in timing, attendance, and seating at meals.

◆ Demonstrate acceptable eating behavior and require that older siblings also set an example.

◆ Do not use food as a comforter or a reward.

◆ Avoid force-feeding or threatening behaviors related to feeding.

◆ Avoid expressions such as "eat for mother."

◆ These guidelines should enable the child's successful transition to self-feeding and the ability to use mealtime for positive social interactions.

Feeding Skills in Infancy and Early Childhood

Motor and Mental Abilities	Interaction	Concerns
Birth to 6 Months		
❖ Sucks	❖ Totally dependent	❖ Incoordination of
❖ Hands to midline	for feeding but may	suck/swallow reflex
❖ Reaches, grasps	initiate oral activity	❖ Spitting excessively
❖ Coordinates suck/		❖ Apathy
swallow reflex		❖ Limited intake
❖ Follows parent		❖ Slow feeding
with eyes		❖ Insatiability
6 to 8 Months		
❖ Sits up	❖ Begins finger-feeding,	❖ Irregularity
❖ Holds objects	eg, hard crackers,	❖ Delay in recognizing
❖ Uses raking grasp	crusty bread	approach of bottle
❖ Vocalizes		or feeding situations
nonspecifically		❖ Choking
8 to 12 Months		
❖ Uses pincer grasp	❖ Self-feeding begins	❖ Messiness
❖ Cruises	❖ Eats from spoon	❖ Bottle in bed
❖ Stands	❖ Plays with food	❖ Poor intake
❖ Walks	❖ Food preference	
❖ May drink from cup	begins	
❖ Vocalizes specifically		
12 to 18 Months		
❖ Climbs, throws	❖ Strong food preferences	❖ Not weaned
❖ Speaks three words	❖ Weaned to cup	❖ Does not finish food
❖ Imitates behaviors	❖ Self-feeding	❖ Decreased appetite
18 to 24 Months		
❖ Well coordinated	❖ Exclusively self-feeding	❖ Picky eater
❖ Autonomous		❖ Pica
❖ Improving verbal		
communication		
24 to 36 Months		
❖ Adept at motor	❖ Social skills at meals	❖ "Bad manners"
skills	developing	❖ Food refusal
❖ Well-developed		
verbal skills		

Suggested Readings

American Academy of Pediatrics. *Feeding Kids Right Isn't Always Easy: Tips for Preventing Food Hassles* (brochure). Elk Grove Village, IL: American Academy of Pediatrics; 1991

Finney JW. Preventing common feeding problems in infants and young children. *Pediatr Clin North Am.* 1986;33:775–788

Nelson K. Feeding problems. In: Parker S, Zuckerman B, eds. *Behavioral and Developmental Pediatrics: A Handbook for Primary Care.* Boston, MA: Little Brown & Co; 1995:143–148

Satter E. *Child of Mine: Feeding With Love and Good Sense.* Palo Alto, CA: Bull Publishing Co; 1991

Temper Tantrums

Tantrums are common in toddlers and preschoolers and can follow minor frustrations or even occur for no obvious reason. Having a temper tantrum is a normal way for young children to express frustration. Tantrums may involve crying and screaming, thrashing, head banging, breath holding, breaking objects, being aggressive toward others, and throwing oneself on the ground. They are a normal part of life and may be considered self-limited developmental manifestations unless they are frequent, violent, prolonged, or persist beyond 4 or 5 years of age.

As young children strive to become more competent and independent, they confront frustrations arising from their own developmental limitations, physical obstacles, and/or restrictions set by others. Because young children have little ability to talk about what they experience, they tend to act out their distress or frustration.

Several factors are believed to predispose children to intense, prolonged, and persisting tantrums:

Predisposing constitutional factors include temperamental factors such as impulsivity and impatience, and developmental factors such as motor and/or cognitive deficits that hamper relationships with people and the ability to negotiate, language delays that prevent the child from expressing anger and frustration, or physical impairments and illnesses that deplete the child's tolerance to stress.

Predisposing parental factors include inconsistent, overly restrictive, or overly indulgent child-rearing patterns. Parents may be threatened by the child's growing independence and, therefore, impose unnecessary and upsetting restrictions and punishments. Other parents who themselves have low frustration tolerances or whose coping resources are depleted due to various pressures (family conflicts, socioeconomic stresses, depression, illness, death, or divorce) may tend to react to the child's increased frustration with inconsistent practices, lack of understanding, anger, and rejection. If parents act in an angry, out-of-control manner, children are likely to imitate them. Tantrum behavior that produces a desired effect for the child has an increased likelihood of recurrence.

Predisposing environmental factors include a physically restrictive, overcrowded, noisy environment with limited space to move and explore, presence of older, aggressive siblings or favored younger ones, competition with peers for territorial rights and toys, and various material privations.

Intervention

Pediatric management of tantrums begins with anticipatory guidance about problem behaviors and patterns of discipline that start in the child's first year. Information about the nature of tantrums, developmental considerations, and the situations that are likely to precipitate tantrums can be provided. Parents need assurance that some tantrum activity is normal, expected, and self-limited. Parents also need advice about how to avoid tantrums and how to handle tantrum behavior should it occur.

To manage tantrums, encourage parents to:

- ◆ Set reasonable limits.

- ◆ Maintain a daily routine.

- ◆ Avoid long outings and visits or take books or other items along to occupy the child.

- ◆ Keep healthful snacks available.

- ◆ Make sure the child is well rested.

- ◆ Distract the child from activities likely to result in a tantrum.

- ◆ Say "no" selectively.

- ◆ Provide children with a predictably nurturant environment with consistent routines, rules, and age-appropriate outlets for behavior.

- ◆ Teach, encourage, and praise desired behaviors.

- ◆ Supervise young children, and avoid, when possible, environmental and situational factors contributing to tantrums. Children can sometimes be redirected from situations likely to lead to trouble.

- ◆ Cue children for potentially difficult transitions from one activity or environment to another.

- ◆ Offer choices to children in order to satisfy their growing need to exert some control (eg, "It's time for your bath. Would you like to walk upstairs or have me carry you?").

- ◆ Encourage expression of frustration and reinforce increased ability of the child to tolerate frustration.

- ◆ Temper tantrums should not be seen as threats to parents. Stressed parents may need reasonable respites from seemingly relentless child demands.

- ◆ Remain calm when dealing with temper tantrums. Modeling self-control increases the likelihood that the child will eventually behave in a similarly composed manner. Violent measures aggravate the problem and are models for violent behaviors.

◆ Emphatically and supportively acknowledge the child's feelings and help the child understand how he or she is feeling. For example, "I am sorry that you are angry, but I can't allow you to throw your toy."

◆ Ignore attention-seeking or demanding tantrums.

◆ Use time-out for disruptive tantrums that cannot be ignored such as those that involve harm to another individual or destruction of property. The child should be restrained or held in a calm and nonreinforcing manner if this is needed; such holding indicates that the parent can provide support and controls when the child needs them most.

◆ Remove the child to a calmer place (such as his or her own room) when the tantrum is too intense to respond to another approach. The removal should be done supportively and not punitively.

◆ Do not give in to the demands of the tantrum or it will increase the likelihood of recurrence.

◆ Allow school-age children to work out their frustration without too much adult interference, providing them with an opportunity to develop their own problem-solving skills and controls.

Frequent, intense temper tantrums may be one of several symptoms indicating significant parent-child conflict or other stresses within the family. Tantrums may become a means for the child to communicate feelings of unhappiness, fear, or discomfort, to obtain attention for needs that are otherwise not fulfilled, or to manipulate parents whose limit-setting practices are inconsistent. Persistent tantrums are a signal of ongoing distress for the child or the family system, and may suggest the need for a consultation with or even referral to a behavioral pediatrician or a mental health professional.

Suggested Readings

American Academy of Pediatrics. *Discipline and Your Child* (brochure). Elk Grove Village, IL: American Academy of Pediatrics; 1998

American Academy of Pediatrics. *Temper Tantrums: a Normal Part of Growing Up* (brochure). Elk Grove Village, IL: American Academy of Pediatrics; 1989

Green M, Palfrey JS, eds. *Bright Futures: Guidelines for Health Supervision of Infants, Children, and Adolescents.* 2nd ed. Arlington, VA: National Center for Education in Maternal and Child Health; 2000

Stein MT. Eighteen months: asserting oneself, a push-pull process. In: Dixon SID, Stein MT. *Encounters With Children — Pediatric Behavior and Development.* 2nd ed. St Louis, MO: Mosby-Yearbook Co; 1992:229–233

Smith EE, Van Tessele. Problems in discipline in early childhood. *Pediatr Clin North Am.* 1982;29:167–176

Sammons W. *I Wanna Do It Myself.* New York, NY: Hyperion Publishing; 1992

Clark L. *The Time-out Solution.* Chicago, IL: Contemporary Books; 1989

Faber A, Mazlish E. *How To Talk So Kids Will Listen.* New York, NY: Avon Press; 1980

Toilet Training

Preparation for toilet training is an important part of pediatric anticipatory guidance. Parents and clinicians find it useful to approach this milestone in the context of overall developmental tasks. Successful toilet training is a reflection of the child's emerging independence and autonomy. Similar to self-feeding, language acquisition, and learning to fall asleep alone, the ability to use a potty seat for elimination strengthens the toddler's sense of self-esteem and independence from parents and other caregivers. Learning to control anal and bladder sphincters and mastering the timing and social skills required to reach the potty seat, to undress, and to eliminate reflect a series of complex developmental tasks that require neurological maturation by the child and attentive, focused guidance by parents.

Parents need to know when to start toilet training, what to expect from their child during the process, what strategies to employ, how long the process is expected to take, and what resources are available to assist them. Because some families try to toilet train their children very early, pediatricians should explore parental attitudes about toilet training during the health care supervision visit at the end of the first year. Discussions about toilet training can take place subsequently during well-child visits until the process is mastered. Written material that explains the process should be made available to parents (eg, AAP brochure on toilet training). Some children and families may be at risk for delays or other difficulties with toilet training, such as children with significant problem behaviors, constipation, or developmental difficulties; more frequent visits to assist these families may prevent future problems of elimination.

It is helpful to explore family attitudes about toilet training, including parental experiences and expectations. Many parents approach toilet training with a good knowledge base and positive feelings about their capacity to train and their child's ability to gain bowel and bladder control.

Other parents are not so certain of themselves or so sensitive to their child's degree of readiness. They may be apprehensive and fearful of setting appropriate limits and concerned about arousing antagonism in their children. These parents may benefit from education, support, and understanding from their pediatrician.

At what age should children be toilet trained? There are no studies comparing different methods or timing of toilet training in terms of efficacy and associated difficulties. In certain cultures parents condition their infants by 6 months of age to achieve a reasonable amount of day and night dryness. Training approaches in the first year of life require physical closeness of mother and infant and place very substantial demands on parents to recognize and respond to the child's indication of elimination needs. In some cultures such training of infants in the first year is done in a relaxed and nurturant fashion. There is no compelling evidence that such early practices lead to later problems with independent toileting. However, it has been observed that for some toddlers, resistant behaviors and anxieties are more likely to occur with early training than thereafter. On the other hand, parents who delay toilet training too long may miss "windows of opportunity" when the child is more receptive to toilet training.

The eventual goal is for children to achieve independent toileting, which cannot occur until certain developmental milestones are achieved. The current consensus among pediatricians is that toilet training should not commence until children show signs of readiness such as an awareness of impending urination or defecation, prolonged involuntary dryness, and some ability to postpone briefly the urge to urinate or defecate. Other physical signs of readiness include the ability to walk easily, pull loose-fitting clothes on and off, and climb on and off a potty chair. These indicators are rarely achieved before 20 to 24 months of age. It is also helpful if children have achieved sufficient responsiveness and understanding to identify body parts, change position at request, imitate simple tasks (such as playing patty-cake), and follow instructions (such as bringing a familiar object or placing one object with another). Behavioral readiness at this age means an increasing tendency toward imitative behaviors, pride in independent skills, a desire to please the parents, and showing a preference for cleanliness.

Toilet training should be as pleasant as possible for both parent and child. The optimal process is a relaxed, unpressured approach based on positive reinforcement and no punishment for accidents. Toilet training should be delayed until signs of readiness appear, usually between 18 and 30 months of age. The importance of timing the initiation of toilet training according to the child's readiness allows the child freedom to master each step according to his or her individual pace, temperament, and behavioral style.

A child-sized potty chair is recommended rather than an adult toilet seat. If an adult toilet is used, adaptations should be made to allow the child to climb on and off easily, sit comfortably, and have adequate foot support. The initial stage involves taking adequate time to allow the child to become familiar with the potty chair. After the child is at ease with and friendly toward the potty chair, the child is introduced to the idea of depositing urine or feces in the potty. Exposure to modeling of toileting activities by older siblings or parents may be useful. Any cooperation or success toward using the potty appropriately is rewarded with praise and encouragement. After the intended idea has been adequately conveyed, the child's diaper is removed at a time when the child is likely to have a bowel movement or urinate. The child is encouraged to sit on the potty; if he or she eliminates successfully, moderate praise or perhaps another small reward is given. It can be helpful to encourage routine sittings on the potty at specified times during the day.

Once the child has demonstrated interest and repeated successes, diapers should no longer be used and training pants can be initiated. "Accidents" are dealt with calmly in a matter-of-fact fashion, without shaming or other punishment. Positive reinforcement and encouragement allow the child to eventually achieve and maintain mastery of the process. From initiation to mastery can take from days to months, depending on the individual child and family situations. With this practice, about 80% of children achieve success at daytime bowel and bladder training by 30 months of age.

The underlying principles of success at any age appear to be consistency, a supportive environment, and appropriate recognition of and response to the child's developmental situation, individual needs, and response to the training.

Practices to Avoid

Many parents will benefit from specific information about practices to avoid in toilet training. Parents should be cautioned about starting too early, during times of extreme stubbornness, or during family stresses (holidays, relocations, new siblings). There should be no battles, punishment, or scolding. It may take several weeks, even months, before toilet training is completed, so parents need to be prepared for "accidents." Other practices to be avoided include prolonged sitting (detention) on the toilet, leaving the child while sitting on the potty, flushing the toilet prematurely, and exhibiting disgust with the waste products.

Toileting Problems

For many parents, reassurance and information will adequately resolve toilet training concerns or difficulties. For others, the assessment and treatment of children with toilet training problems often involve addressing complex parental issues. It is important to determine whether the toileting difficulty is an isolated problem or one of several areas of conflicts for the child and family. Complicating child or family characteristics may need to be addressed. In order to understand the situation, it is often helpful to have parents describe specific scenarios. The parents' perception of the reasons for the difficulty and their emotional reactions to it need to be addressed and acknowledged.

A patient, sensitive, empathic approach by the physician toward parents helps model a patient, sensitive, and empathic approach by parents to the child. Circumstances that interfere with the ability of the parents to guide the child appropriately need to be discussed and addressed.

Toileting Resistance

The guiding principles for parents faced with a toddler who resists toilet training are the same as those for working with other resistant behavior; reward positive achievements and deemphasize undesirable behaviors. Reducing emphasis on toileting failures deflates power from the symptom and is a relief to the parents. When incentives for proper toileting are presented and parental investment in success is deemphasized, the chances for success are significantly increased. Reminders to the child about toileting should stop, and responsibility for toileting should be given to the child. Significant constipation should be treated medically. Many parents of children who persistently resist toilet training benefit from counseling regarding general behavioral issues as well as toileting issues.

Suggested Readings

American Academy of Pediatrics. *Bed-wetting* (brochure). Elk Grove Village, IL: American Academy of Pediatrics; 1996

American Academy of Pediatrics. *Toilet Training* (brochure). Elk Grove Village, IL: American Academy of Pediatrics; 1993

Brazelton TB. A child-oriented approach to toilet training. *Pediatrics.* 1962;29:121–128

deVries MW, deVries MR. Cultural relativity of toilet training readiness: a perspective from East Africa. *Pediatrics.* 1977;60:170–172

Luxem M, Christophersen E. Behavioral training in early childhood: research, practice, and implications.*J Dev Behav Pediatr.* 1994;15:370–378

Howe AC, Walker CE. Behavioral management of toilet training, enuresis, and encopresis. *Pediatr Clin North Am.* 1992;39:413–432

Ross Growth and Development Series. *Developing Toilet Habits.* Columbus, OH: Ross Laboratories; 1986

Schmitt BD. Toilet training refusal: avoid the battle and win the war. *Contemp Pediatr.* 1987;32–50

Sleep Problems

Sleep is a highly organized physiologic process that is influenced by the care-giving environment. Putting a child to bed and helping the child to sleep through the night are important tasks. Most children in our culture need to develop internal controls to stay asleep. The role of the parents is to facilitate this process.

Sleep patterns and nighttime behaviors among infants and young children vary and develop in response to individual characteristics and environmental factors. Reluctance to go to sleep and night waking are common occurrences. For some parents these sleep behaviors become a problem. It is generally much easier to prevent sleep problems than it is to treat them later. Thus, information about sleep should be part of anticipatory guidance for the parents of infants and young children.

Sleep States

Normal sleep is composed of two distinct states, rapid eye movement (REM) and nonrapid eye movement (NREM) sleep. REM sleep is a lighter stage of sleep and is characterized by an irregular pulse and respiratory rate, body twitches, suppression of muscle tone, rapid eye movements, and dreams. NREM sleep, varying from drowsiness to deep sleep, is a more physiologically organized state, characterized by regular pulse and respiratory rate and minimal body move-ments. During the deepest stages of NREM sleep, the body is relaxed and the mind free of thoughts and dreams, and breathing is slow and regular. Children are difficult to awaken during this time.

A sleep cycle consists of NREM sleep followed by REM sleep. Sleep cycles last just under an hour in infants and about twice that long in adults. The propor-tionate amount of time spent in active REM sleep diminishes as the infant becomes older. Infants may normally achieve a state of quiet wakefulness at the end of a sleep cycle, but can learn to return to sleep through self-quieting behaviors. Increasing sleep duration is a reflection of infant central nervous system maturation and the ability to suppress arousal.

Developmental Issues

Neonates and infants

Parents should be encouraged to carry and hold their babies frequently during the daytime. A differential responsiveness from parents during daytime and night-time teaches a child that nighttime is for sleeping and daytime is for wakefulness.

219

Babies who are allowed to sleep for many consecutive hours during the day may have trouble sleeping for long consecutive periods at night. Parents should be encouraged to help children learn to settle themselves to sleep without external assistance such as holding, rocking, or feeding. Parents should be made aware that frequent daytime feeders are likely to want to be frequent nighttime feeders. The number of nighttime feedings will be more likely to gradually decrease if feeding intervals during the day are adequately spaced and if nighttime feedings are performed in as short a time as possible. By a few months of age, many infants are learning how to self-comfort and self-induce sleep.

By this age it is sensible to have the baby sleep in a room separate from the parents. The volume of feedings and reinforcing attention given at night should be less than that which occurs during daytime feedings. Parents should encourage their children to learn self-soothing behaviors rather than to become dependent on external parental interventions at bedtime and during the night. When older infants awaken and cry during the night, they often can soothe themselves or be comforted with soothing behaviors and words instead of feeding. Parental contact with infants in the middle of the night should be brief and quieting in order that infants learn to go back to sleep on their own.

By the middle of the first year of life, many children are anxious about separation from their parents. A stuffed animal, doll, blanket, or other security object can give added comfort to the child when going to sleep and when the child awakens during the night. Consistently pleasant and predictable bedtime routines and rituals help promote good sleep habits. Children who spend time with their parents before going to bed feel more secure.

The infant's environment should be the same upon falling asleep as it will be when the infant has normal physiological awakenings during the night. For this reason, babies should not be given bottles to take to bed with them. Bedtime bottles or pacifiers can become part of an infant's sleep associations, which will be difficult for an infant to re-create in order to return to sleep during the night and can lead to nursing bottle caries.

Toddlers and preschoolers

The separation issues that are commonly seen in toddlers and preschoolers have an impact on a child's sleep. During this stage, children want to be with their parents. Bedtime routines, rituals, transitional objects, consistency, and reassurances from the parents are important. Children with nighttime fears should be calmly reassured. Parents should be told of the importance of appropriate sleep behaviors for the child.

Autonomy issues can also be extremely important for toddlers and preschoolers. Clear expectations, reinforcing desired behaviors, and offering choices to the child can be helpful in establishing good sleep habits. The pediatrician should be aware of whether bedtime difficulties or repeated awakenings are an isolated problem or part of a larger behavior management problem for the family. Parents may need help with general behavior management techniques in order to improve both daytime and nighttime behaviors. Management of sleep problems involves understanding the child's temperament, psychosocial situation, and parental attitudes and feelings.

Anticipatory guidance about sleep should be part of well-child visits in the preschool period, including discussions during office visits and literature made available to parents. Families who are experiencing sleep problems should receive specific information about how to deal with them. Sleep problems such as frequent night wakings or resistance to bedtime that reflect parent-child interactive difficulties should be addressed along with appropriate attention given to individual situational issues for the family.

Night terrors

Night terrors (pavor nocturnus) are categorized as a disorder of arousal occurring during a transition from stage IV, NREM sleep to REM sleep. Night terrors occur with greatest frequency in preschool and early school age children. Similar brief confusional arousals may occur in younger children. Night terrors usually occur within a couple of hours of falling asleep. Children can cry inconsolably and appear terrified, confused, and glassy-eyed. Autonomic activity, characterized by sweating, tachycardia, and tachypnea, is common. Children do not appear to realize that anyone is with them. They appear frightened but cannot be awakened or comforted. Parents need to be reassured that these events are short-lived and that they do not necessarily indicate an emotional disturbance or response to overwhelming daytime stresses. Because children with night terrors return to sleep spontaneously and have no later memory of the episodes, parents should be encouraged to protect the child against injury during the episode and to calmly try to help the child return to normal sleep. Parents may need reassurance that the child is not disturbed or suffering. Frequent night terrors suggest exploration into the child's life situation. Overtiredness should be avoided. There is evidence that prompted awakenings can help reduce frequent night terrors.

Sleep walking

Sleep walking, also considered a disorder of arousal, is common and tends to run in families. It may occur several times a night. Parents should be advised to remove hazards in the child's room, lock outside doors, and block stairways. There is no need to wake the child; just lead the child back to bed. A regular sleep schedule and dealing with stressful issues may help prevent sleep walking.

Talking in one's sleep is considered another disorder of arousal. No treatment is needed.

Nightmares

Night terrors that occur in a transitional state from deep to lighter sleep need to be differentiated from nightmares that occur during REM sleep. An occasional nightmare is common. Unlike the child with night terrors, the child with night-mares can recall the dream and may be fearful about returning to sleep. Children who have nightmares need soothing reassurance when they awaken. Children need to know that they were having a bad dream but that in reality they are safe. Children can be encouraged to talk about their bad dream during the day and assisted in dealing with difficult feelings. Children should be shielded from unnecessarily frightening or anxiety-producing situations, including television exposure that may be upsetting. Occasionally nightmares are signals of significant stresses that should be investigated and addressed by parents and professionals if needed.

Suggested Readings

American Academy of Pediatrics. *Guide to Your Child's Sleep.* New York, NY: Villard Books; 1999

American Academy of Pediatrics. *Sleep Problems in Children.* Elk Grove Village, IL: American Academy of Pediatrics; 1994

Cuthbertson J, Schevill S. *Helping Your Child Steep Through the Night.* New York, NY: Main Street Books; 1985

Ferber R. *Solve Your Child's Sleep Problems.* New York, NY: Simon and Schuster; 1985

Green M, Palfrey JS, eds. *Bright Futures: Guidelines for Health Supervision of Infants, Children, and Adolescents.* 2nd ed. Arlington, VA: National Center for Education in Maternal and Child Health; 2000

Individual Differences

Most books on child care describe the development and treatment of the "average" child and only mention the variations of normal. Children display many kinds of normal variations. Differences in height, body type, and coloring of hair, eyes, and skin are well known. There are also normal differences in development and cognitive functions as well as individual differences in temperament or behavioral style.

A child's temperament is his or her behavioral style or the way the child experiences and reacts to environmental influences.

Temperament is derived primarily from genetic influences but also from the psychosocial environment and other factors such as the child's physical health and development. Temperament is weakly to moderately stable in the early months of life and becomes increasingly consistent as the child gets older.

A child's temperament in turn affects his or her behavior, development, and interactions with parents. Temperament may be a source of concern for parents because certain characteristics of their child's temperament may complicate their efforts at caregiving and discipline.

The characteristics of temperament listed below are from Chess and Thomas (1986). Numerous other conceptualizations have been proposed by other researchers.

- *activity:* the amount of physical motion during sleep, play, dressing, and bathing
- *rhythmicity:* the regularity of physiological functions such as hunger, sleep, and elimination, including predictability of habits in an older child
- *approach/withdrawal:* the nature of initial responses to new people, places, foods, toys, and procedures
- *adaptability:* the ease or difficulty with which reactions to stimuli can be modified
- *intensity:* the energy level of responses regardless of quality or direction
- *mood:* the amount of pleasant and friendly behavior or unpleasant and unfriendly behavior in various situations
- *persistence/attention span:* the length of time particular activities are pursued by the child
- *distractibility:* the effectiveness of extraneous stimuli in interfering with ongoing behaviors
- *sensory threshold:* the amount of stimulation, such as sounds or light, necessary to evoke discernible responses

Frequently several of the above-mentioned characteristics are clustered in a particular child. For example, the cluster of low rhythmicity, low approach, low adaptability, high intensity, and negative mood has been related to behavior problems. The cluster of high activity, low persistence/attention span, and high distractibility may be associated with lower scholastic achievement.

Discussions with parents about their child's temperament often improve their general understanding. Identification of the specific child's temperament profile helps to define his or her contribution to the interactions and helps parents to modify their caregiving techniques to minimize the stresses to their child.

When a behavioral problem has developed, knowledge of the child's temperament may help to explain the origins of the condition and guide the clinician and parents in future management.

A child's temperament may become a clinical problem if (1) a "poor fit" between the child's temperament and the social environment creates misunderstanding or conflicts; (2) the temperamental characteristics become augmented into a non-adaptive coping style, such as when low adaptability turns into rigidity or low initial approach develops into excessive avoidance of novelty; or (3) parents are concerned even if the child is not noticeably dysfunctional.

Referral of a child to a behavioral pediatrician or mental health professional is usually not necessary or appropriate for variations in temperament, but may be helpful if moderate or severe secondary behavior problems persist.

Suggested Readings for Professionals

Chess S, Thomas A. *Temperament in Clinical Practice.* New York, NY: Guilford; 1986

Carey WB, McDevitt SC. *Coping with Children's Temperament: A Guide for Professionals.* New York, NY: Basic Books; 1995

Suggested Readings for Parents

Green M, Palfrey JS, eds. *Bright Futures: Guidelines for Health Supervision of Infants, Children, and Adolescents.* 2nd ed. Arlington, VA: National Center for Education in Maternal and Child Health; 2000

Kurcinka MS. *Raising Your Spirited Child: A Guide for Parents Whose Child Is More Intense, Sensitive, Perceptive, Persistent, Energetic.* New York, NY: Harper Collins; 1991

Turecki S, Tonner L. *The Difficult Child.* Revised Edition. New York, NY: Bantam Books; 1989

Effective Discipline

Discipline refers to the structure that parents create to teach their children how they are expected to behave. The term *discipline* is often used in a much more limited fashion, to refer only to *punishment.* Punishment, however, is only a very small part of the total parenting environment that helps children to feel safe, capable, and lovable and helps parents to feel effective.

Pediatricians are often the most accessible professionals in contact with children and families during the preschool period and thus have the opportunity (and therefore also the responsibility) to help parents in their efforts to provide the best possible context for growth. Because effective discipline is central to the structure of the family, its discussion should be a part of every health supervision visit. Table I provides some guidelines regarding discussions about how discipline can be woven usefully into the context of health supervision visits.

Preventive strategies

It is important to remember that each child exists in the context of a complex family that is an interactive and interdependent system. Parents generally want to do what is best for their children. They may be limited by inadequate knowledge of appropriate strategies and techniques, depression or anxiety, overwhelming challenges of their own life situations, anger, or psychopathology. Parents rely primarily on their intuition and their own childhood experiences to guide their parenting actions. Pediatricians need to provide support, direction, and, occasionally, specific guidance.

Several specific strategies help children feel loved and capable. The first strategy includes a short but defined period of time that each parent schedules with each child. During this time, each parent and child interact in pleasurable activities without interruptions.

Parents also should attend to and praise their children liberally when they are playing appropriately, relating well with an adult or a child, trying to be helpful, or making any attempt to do what the parent asks. The most effective praise takes the form of short, direct verbal messages, preferably referring directly to the parent's feelings rather than the child's behavior. Nonverbal messages are powerful as well, such as a hug, a smile, or a pat on the back.

A third strategy involves encouraging children to take part in appropriate decisions, teaching them that they are responsible for their behavior. Choices must be appropriate to the child's developmental abilities, and parents should be sure that all the options offered are acceptable to them.

Shaping the behavior of children

Increasing desirable behavior

All behavior is learned, shaped primarily by its consequences. Behaviors that are rewarded or reinforced are likely to continue and even increase in frequency. Reinforcement provided by parents may be intentional or inadvertent, and the behavior reinforced may be desirable or undesirable (Tables 2 and 3).

Examples of intentional reinforcement of behavior include a parent's praise for appropriate play or accomplishment of a task, a planned gift, or a joint activity contingent on the child's completion of a particular assignment. Inadvertent rewards for good behavior may include a smile on the mother's face as she watches her child create a high tower and take pleasure in knocking it down or having the child overhear a parent speaking with pride about school accomplishments. Unfortunately, however, inadvertent reinforcement also occurs in relation to **undesirable** behavior. A child who receives a cookie to head off a temper tantrum or is fed each time he or she awakens during the night is receiving unintentional rewards for behavior the parents would rather discourage. Similarly, some attempts by parents to punish their children's unacceptable behavior may be in some way reinforcing the behavior rather than discouraging it. Some negative attention from parents may be better than none at all; "yelling" is at least intense interaction, though not encouraged.

Table 1.
Recommended Contexts for Discussions
About Discipline at Various Ages

Age	Contexts to Frame Discussions About Discipline
1–4 mo	sleeping and eating schedules/routines
6–9 mo	rules to ensure safety of environment
12–18 mo	emerging autonomy and independence
2 y	toileting, perhaps new sibling
3 y	entering preschool
4 y	household chores
5 y	entering more formal school setting
6–12 y	increasing peer activities and orientation
Adolescence	curfews, guidelines for alcohol use, driving, sexual behavior

Decreasing undesirable behavior

Children learn faster and better by being rewarded for good behavior than by being punished for bad behavior. Nevertheless, because all children at some time behave in inappropriate ways, their parents must find a way to indicate that these behaviors are not acceptable and to decrease their frequency. Reinforcement for the behaviors can be withdrawn (ignoring), and/or they can result in an unpleasant consequence, either naturally occurring or imposed by adults in the environment (punishment).

Punishment can take two forms: (1) privileges or pleasurable activities can be denied, or (2) painful, uncomfortable, or undesirable circumstances or activities can be imposed. Examples of the restriction of privileges include decreasing the amount of time the child may watch television, decreasing the number of books a parent will read at bedtime, or not allowing the child to eat dessert with the family. Examples of the imposition of undesirable circumstances include requiring certain chores to be done or imposing separation of the child from the activities of the family, such as "time-out."

The most powerful punishments are consequences that occur **naturally** as a result of the child's behavior, eg, dawdling in the morning results in being late for school; if a child does not eat at mealtime, he or she may be hungry by the time it is bedtime. Parents need only refrain from interfering with the natural consequences that follow the child's behavior. Parents also can create negative consequences that follow **logically**. Scribbling on the wall might result in not

Table 2.
Basic Rules for Effective Discipline

◆ Reward behavior you like	Rewards can be tangible or symbolic. Reward should be immediate. Hugs and praise are powerful rewards.
◆ Use natural and logical consequences as your ally	*Natural* consequences are what would happen if you did nothing. *Logical* consequences are those you impose as a reasonable outcome of the specific behavior.
◆ Punish behavior you do not like	Take away something the child values, or impose something the child dislikes. Punishment should be immediate. Frequent small punishments are more effective than occasional extensive punishments. Spanking is effective only for the moment and has undesirable side effects.

Table 3.
Common Pitfalls Leading to Ineffective Discipline

- Inadvertent rewarding of undesirable behavior
- Failure to notice and reward desirable behavior
- Insufficient "time-in"
- Inconsistent rules from day to day, situation to situation
- Too many punishable behaviors

allowing the child to use crayons for a week or in the assignment of washing the walls; if toys are not put away by a prescribed time, they are removed for several days. Some unacceptable behaviors require parents to create a more contrived intervention. For example, hitting or biting does not result in any immediate, logical, or natural negative consequence; thus, an extrinsic punishment needs to be imposed. For maximal effectiveness, punishments such as time-out should be instituted in a planned, carefully specified manner after they have been described to the child. Table 4 lists strategies to prevent undesirable behavior.

Although opinions vary among pediatricians, spanking and other forms of physical punishment are not advisable. Although spanking may at first appear effective as a result of the child's surprise, pain, and fear, long term it is seldom effective and is utilized at risk of considerable negative consequences.

- Spanking provides a model of a type of behavior that parents generally do not allow for the child; how can young children understand that their parents may hit them while they themselves are punished for hitting other children?

- Physical punishment undermines the effective, cooperative, and nurturing relationship parents hope to have with their children. Children who are spanked may learn aggressive and violent forms of conflict resolution based on power and strength, and they are more likely as adults to be depressed, use alcohol, have more anger, and hit their children and spouses. Children, like adults, feel violated, shamed, hurt, and angry when they are hit.

- Spanking lessens the effectiveness of other disciplinary measures; eventually its impact is lost as well.

Table 4.
Preventive Strategies

1. Empowerment of parents

2. Discipline = **rules** and **consequences**

3. Praise and attend

4. Time alone

5. Effective choices

◆ Most parents are reluctant to resort to spanking. They don't like to hurt their children, and they often recognize that spanking is effective only at the moment and does not inform future behavior. As a result of their uncertainty and delays in instituting appropriate consequences for undesirable behavior, parents often feel ineffective, angry, and frustrated.

It is very important to remember that *punishment* is *never enough*. At best, punishment only teaches children what behavior is *not* acceptable, but cannot teach what behavior is desirable. Effective discipline results when the environment allows children to feel *safe* by virtue of predictable rules and consequences, *lovable* as a result of adequate attention and praise, and *capable* of making decisions and taking responsibility for their own behavior.

Suggested Readings for Professionals

Christophersen ER. Discipline. *Pediatr Clin North Am.* 1992;39:395–411

Friedman SB, Schonberg SK. The short- and long-term consequences of corporal punishment. *Pediatrics.* 1996;98(suppl):803–806

Howard BJ. Discipline in early childhood. *Pediatr Clin North Am.* 1991;38:1351–1369

Larzelere RE. Moderate spanking: model or deterrent of children's aggression in the family? *J Family Violence.* 1986;1:27–36

McCormick KF. Attitudes of primary care physicians toward corporal punishment. *JAMA.* 1992;267:3161–3165

Schmitt BD. Discipline: rules and consequences. *Contemp Pediatr.* 1991;65–69

Smith EE, Van Tassel E. Problems of discipline in early childhood. *Pediatr Clin North Am.* 1982;29:167–176

Suggested Readings for Parents

American Academy of Pediatrics. *Discipline and Your Child* (brochure). Elk Grove Village, IL: American Academy of Pediatrics; 1998

American Academy of Pediatrics, Family Communications. *What Do You Do With the Mad That You Feel?* (brochure). Elk Grove Village, IL: American Academy of Pediatrics; 1997

American Academy of Pediatrics. *Thumbs, Fingers, and Pacifiers* (brochure). Elk Grove Village, IL: American Academy of Pediatrics; 1997

Brazelton TB. *Touchpoints: Your Child's Emotional and Behavioral Development.* Reading, MA: Addison-Wesley Publishing Co; 1992

Clark L. *The Time-Out Solution: A Parent's Guide for Handling Everyday Behavior Problems.* Chicago, IL: Contemporary Books; 1989

Dreikurs R. *Children: The Challenge.* New York, NY: Duell, Sloan & Pearce; 1964

Dreikurs R, Grey LA. *Parent's Guide to Child Discipline.* New York, NY: Hawthorn Books; 1970

Faber A, Mazlish E. *How to Talk So Kids Will Listen and Listen So Kids Will Talk.* New York, NY: Avon Books; 1982

Green M, Palfrey JS, eds. *Bright Futures: Guidelines for Health Supervision of Infants, Children, and Adolescents.* 2nd ed. Arlington, VA: National Center for Education in Maternal and Child Health; 2000

Self-Comforting Behaviors

A number of self-comforting or self-stimulating behaviors that are of interest to pediatricians and parents, including thumb-sucking, head banging, body rocking, and similar others, are seen often in normally developing children. Pediatricians can play an important role in offering reassurance to parents. At the same time, the pediatrician should be able to determine when these behaviors have become deviant and therefore require closer vigilance or intervention. Physicians should provide pediatric counseling or appropriate referral if such behaviors persist into school years or interfere with social interactions because of the intensity or type of the behavior.

The use of pacifiers, for example, is widespread and frequently becomes a concern for many parents and some health care professionals. For many infants, however, sucking on a pacifier may be quite healthful; the need for sucking varies greatly among babies. Other related behaviors such as thumb-sucking, fingering, fingering of hair or ear lobes, body rocking, head rolling or banging, masturbation or frequent handling of the genitalia, and even sucking on the toes are seen in otherwise normally developing children. These behaviors also may be observed in association with blindness, mental retardation, or in children with emotional disturbances seeking relief or communicating tension.

Children's Factors

Pediatricians should expect to hear about, and should inquire about, self-stimulating behaviors. Just as children differ in temperament, they vary in their need for tension relief. The manner of such release, whether through rubbing the nose with a blanket, rocking, or sucking, probably has multiple determinants. Even fetuses have been observed to suck their fingers or thumbs. The use of body stimulation for the relief of tension is more common in younger children than in older children.

Parents' Perspective

Just as infants vary in their abilities and expressions, so do parents. Although one parent might view an infant's genital play negatively, another might view the behavior as evidence of "growing up" or normal maturation. Parents are products of their own upbringing, and their attitudes about their child's self-comforting behaviors reflect this. Parents who are not concerned and do not react negatively to the behaviors may casually distract the baby from the behavior. Other parents may become tense and further reinforce the behaviors by their own anxiety, for example, by pulling the child's thumb from his or her mouth or expressing anger regarding the use of pacifiers in public.

Pediatric Management

The pediatrician's understanding of the frequency and normalcy of self-comforting behaviors in young children will help in advising parents. Questions to parents about the child's interest and awareness of body parts may lead to discussions of parental concern about masturbation and other activities. The pediatrician needs to be knowledgeable about normal child development and respect the cultural background of the family.

When self-stimulating behaviors persist into the school years or interfere with normal social interactions (eg, the 6-year-old child who masturbates in school) and are of great concern to the parents, a more in-depth assessment of parent-child interaction is indicated. However, even older children under stress may, for brief periods of time, regress to self-comforting behaviors. For the most part, such behaviors are part of normal human development. Pediatric counseling should be reassuring to parents. In-depth assessment and counseling, however, may need to be provided by a behavioral pediatrician or a mental health professional under some circumstances. The physician must consider parental attitudes and family culture during counseling. When the pediatrician is following infants or older children at risk for developmental disabilities, it is possible that self-comforting behaviors may manifest a disability; however, a medical etiology should not be overlooked, especially in children who have communication difficulties. Head banging in a child with trisomy 21, for example, could be a behavioral manifestation of a sinus infection or headaches. Poor social interaction and intense body rocking may indicate autism.

Suggested Reading

American Academy of Pediatrics. *Thumbs, Fingers, and Pacifiers* (brochure). Elk Grove Village, IL: American Academy of Pediatrics; 1997

Parental Stress and the Child at Risk

Optimal physical and psychological development of infants and children is influenced by the availability of nurturing parents who can provide attentive care, protection, love, guidance, and discipline. If parents are unable to provide consistent and contingent caregiving, their children are at increased risk for physical, behavioral, and emotional disorders. Pediatricians are in a unique position to recognize the manifestations of stressors in parenting, evaluate the risks involved, and determine the necessary interventions. Health supervision in pediatrics includes identifying factors that create risk for physical, developmental, or psychosocial disorders. When the pediatrician determines that a child is experiencing disturbed parenting, frequent follow up, reassessment, early intervention, and parent support may be necessary to strengthen the child's protective resources and improve the quality of parenting. It is important to refrain from quick assumptions and judgments that may interfere in an effective partnership with parents. The most valuable contribution to this partnership is the pediatrician's ability to listen and offer nonjudgmental support on behalf of the child.

Recognizing the Risks

Pediatricians may observe evidence of difficulties in the family system as they assess the parents, the child, and the interactions among them. Some of the factors that stress parents and can result in increased risk for children are shown in Table 1. Manifestations may include excessive parental anxiety, depression, hostility, drug dependency, frequent need for social or economic support services, marital conflict, and irresponsible parenting.

Table 1.
Parental Characteristics That Place Children at Risk

• *Individual Parent Illness or Vulnerability*	• *Excessive Child-Rearing Responsibilities*
✧ Chronic physical or mental illness	✧ Chronically ill or disabled child
✧ Mental retardation or education deficiencies	✧ Large family
	✧ Multiple birth
✧ Personality disorders	✧ Difficult temperament in the child
✧ Alcoholism or other drug abuse and addiction	
• *Lack of Social or Economic Support Systems*	
✧ Poverty	
✧ Conflictual marriage	
✧ Unavailable social support	
✧ Limited child care resources	

The child may show signs of abuse and neglect or, being reared with more subtle and less damaging parenting dysfunctions, may present with physical, developmental, or behavioral problems. Table 2 presents examples of common findings in stressed family systems, although they are not the only indications of these difficulties.

Pediatricians may also observe parent-child interactions with specific reference to issues of attachment-detachment and autonomy-control. For example, disturbances in attachment may be evidenced by parental apathy, inattentiveness to their child, impatience with the child's demands, or an overanxious response to separation experiences. In addition, observations of the methods and styles of discipline may identify difficulties with setting limits, manifested by excessive punitiveness or overpermissiveness.

Table 2.
Common Findings Suggestive of Parenting Dysfunction

* *Birth to 6 Months*
  * Overanxious or depressed parent
  * Aloof or self-absorbed parent
  * Difficulty in adjusting to parenting demands
  * Frequent nonillness pediatric calls
  * Apathetic baby
  * Feeding problems
  * Nonorganic failure to thrive

* *6 to 18 Months*
  * Inattentive or apathetic parent
  * Inappropriate parental expectations of behavior and development
  * Excessive prohibitions, inconsistent or inappropriate discipline
  * Frequent nonillness pediatric visits
  * Extreme sleep problems
  * Temper tantrums, child abuse
  * Excessive fearfulness or clinginess in nonstressful situations
  * Developmental delay
  * Failure to thrive

* *18 Months to 3 Years*
  * Language and developmental delay
  * Extreme separation difficulties
  * Unyielding opposition
  * Excessive fearfulness and clinging
  * Out-of-control behavior
  * Excessive aggression or destructiveness
  * Repeated injuries and accidents

* *4 to 6 Years*
  * Sleep difficulties
  * Somatic complaints
  * Difficulty with separation and transitions to school
  * Encopresis or daytime and secondary enuresis
  * Excessive parental demands
  * Excessive struggles with cooperation
  * Hyperactivity
  * Vulnerable child syndrome
  * Cruelty to animals
  * Aggressive behaviors (fighting, lying, stealing)
  * Depression, withdrawal, and apathy
  * Psychosocial dwarfism

Parental psychopathology increases the vulnerability of children to later difficulties; recurrent or chronic parental physical illness may place children at increased risk for emotional disturbances, especially when parents exhibit long-standing abnormality of personality. Children of parents who are depressed or psychotic have an increased risk of clinical depression, attention-deficit disorders, and separation problems. Children of overprotective parents may be at increased risk for neurotic and depressive disorders.

Pediatric Intervention

When pediatricians identify children or families at risk, they should recommend appropriate interventions to strengthen the family's resources. Interventions might include referral for individual psychotherapy, family therapy, psychopharmacologic therapy, behavior management training, parenting education, alcohol or other drug treatment, or social services. In the most severe cases, child protective custody may be necessary.

Because of the protective factors of some children, such as their genetic inheritance, temperament, age, coping skills, and previous experience, they are less vulnerable to the negative consequences of dysfunctional systems. When a child has a significant relationship with another healthy adult, the developmental impact of a disturbed parent is lessened. In addition, when family disruption, discord, or conflict is reduced, the child's risk is often reduced. Intervention efforts specifically for the child, in addition to stabilizing the family environment and supporting the significant adults involved with the child, may include developmental intervention programs, child care, preschool programs, and after-school programs. If the pediatrician believes the child to be particularly vulnerable, recommendations for child therapy may be indicated.

Suggested Readings for Professionals

Anthony EJ. The syndrome of the psychologically invulnerable child. In: *The Child and His Family: Children at Psychiatric Risk.* Vol 3. New York, NY: John Wiley and Sons; 1974

Green M, Palfrey JS, eds. *Bright Futures: Guidelines for Health Supervision of Infants, Children, and Adolescents.* 2nd ed. Arlington, VA: National Center for Education in Maternal and Child Health; 2000

Parker G. *Parental Overprotection: A Risk Factor in Psychosocial Development.* New York, NY: Grune and Stratton; 1983

Rutter M. *Children of Sick Parents: An Environmental and Psychiatric Study.* Vol 16. Maudsley Monographs, London, England: Oxford University Press; 1966

Weissman M, Prusoff B, Gammon G, et al. Psychopathology in the children (ages 6–18) of depressed and normal parents. *J Am Acad Child Psychiatry.* 1984;23:78–84

Appendix A

Recommendations for Preventive Pediatric Health Care (RE9939)

Committee on Practice and Ambulatory Medicine

Each child and family is unique; therefore, these **Recommendations for Preventive Pediatric Health Care** are designed for the care of children who are receiving competent parenting, have no manifestations of any important health problems, and are growing and developing in satisfactory fashion. **Additional visits may become necessary** if circumstances suggest variations from normal.

These guidelines represent a consensus by the Committee on Practice and Ambulatory Medicine in consultation with national committees and sections of the American Academy of Pediatrics. The Committee emphasizes the great importance of **continuity of care** in comprehensive health supervision and the need to avoid **fragmentation of care.**

AGE[5]	INFANCY[4]								EARLY CHILDHOOD[4]						MIDDLE CHILDHOOD[4]				ADOLESCENCE[4]										
	PRENATAL[1]	NEWBORN[2]	2-4d[3]	By 1mo	2mo	4mo	6mo	9mo	12mo	15mo	18mo	24mo	3y	4y	5y	6y	8y	10y	11y	12y	13y	14y	15y	16y	17y	18y	19y	20y	21y
HISTORY Initial/Interval	●	●	●	●	●	●	●	●	●	●	●	●	●	●	●	●	●	●	●	●	●	●	●	●	●	●	●	●	●
MEASUREMENTS Height and Weight		●	●	●	●	●	●	●	●	●	●	●	●	●	●	●	●	●	●	●	●	●	●	●	●	●	●	●	●
Head Circumference		●	●	●	●	●	●	●	●	●	●	●																	
Blood Pressure													●	●	●	●	●	●	●	●	●	●	●	●	●	●	●	●	●
SENSORY SCREENING Vision		S		S	S	S	S	S	S	S	S	S	O[6]	O	O	O	O	O	S	O	S	S	O	S	S	O	S	S	S
Hearing		O[7]		S	S	S	S	S	S	S	S	S	O	O	O	O	O	O	S	O	S	S	O	S	S	O	S	S	S
DEVELOPMENTAL/ BEHAVIORAL ASSESSMENT[8]		●	●	●	●	●	●	●	●	●	●	●	●	●	●	●	●	●	●	●	●	●	●	●	●	●	●	●	●
PHYSICAL EXAMINATION[9]		●	●	●	●	●	●	●	●	●	●	●	●	●	●	●	●	●	●	●	●	●	●	●	●	●	●	●	●
PROCEDURES-GENERAL[10] Hereditary/Metabolic Screening[11]		●	←→																										
Immunization[12]		●		●	●	●	●		●	●	●			●	●				●→			←●→							
Hematocrit or Hemoglobin[13]								←●→											★	★									
Urinalysis															●														
PROCEDURES-PATIENTS AT RISK Lead Screening[16]							★	▼	▼	★	★	★	★	★	★	★	★	★											
Tuberculin Test[17]									★			★	★	★	★	★	★	★	★	★	★	★	★	★	★	★	★	★	★
Cholesterol Screening[18]												★	★	★	★	★	★	★	★	★	★	★	★	★	★	★	★	★	★
STD Screening[19]																			★	★	★	★	★	★	★	★	★	★	★
Pelvic Exam[20]																			★	★	★	★	★	★	★	★	★	★[20]	★
ANTICIPATORY GUIDANCE[21] Injury Prevention[22]		●	●	●	●	●	●	●	●	●	●	●	●	●	●	●	●	●	●	●	●	●	●	●	●	●	●	●	●
Violence Prevention[23]		●	●	●	●	●	●	●	●	●	●	●	●	●	●	●	●	●	●	●	●	●	●	●	●	●	●	●	●
Sleep Positioning Counseling[24]		●	●	●	●	●	←→																						
Nutrition Counseling[25]		●	●	●	●	●	●	●	●	●	●	●	●	●	●	●	●	●	●	●	●	●	●	●	●	●	●	●	●
DENTAL REFERRAL[26]												▼	●																

1. A prenatal visit is recommended for parents who are at high risk, for first-time parents, and for those who request a conference. The prenatal visit should include anticipatory guidance, pertinent medical history, and a discussion of benefits of breastfeeding and planned method of feeding per AAP statement "The Prenatal Visit" (1996).
2. Every infant should have a newborn evaluation after birth. Breastfeeding should be encouraged and instruction and support offered. Every breastfeeding infant should have an evaluation 48-72 hours after discharge from the hospital to include weight, formal breastfeeding evaluation, encouragement, and instruction as recommended in the AAP statement "Breastfeeding and the Use of Human Milk" (1997).
3. For newborns discharged in less than 48 hours after delivery per AAP statement "Hospital Stay for Healthy Term Newborns" (1995).
4. Developmental, psychosocial, and chronic disease issues for children and adolescents may require frequent counseling and treatment visits separate from preventive care visits.
5. If a child comes under care for the first time at any point on the schedule, or if any items are not accomplished at the suggested age, the schedule should be brought up to date at the earliest possible time.
6. If the patient is uncooperative, rescreen within 6 months.
7. All newborns should be screened per the AAP Task Force on Newborn and Infant Hearing statement, "Newborn and Infant Hearing Loss: Detection and Intervention" (1999).
8. By history and appropriate physical examination; if suspicious, by specific objective developmental testing. Parenting skills should be fostered at every visit.
9. At each visit, a complete physical examination is essential, with infant totally unclothed, older child undressed and suitably draped.
10. These may be modified, depending upon entry point into schedule and individual need.
11. Metabolic screening (eg, thyroid, hemoglobinopathies, PKU, galactosemia) should be done according to state law.
12. Schedule(s) per the Committee on Infectious Diseases, published annually in the January edition of Pediatrics. Every visit should be an opportunity to update and complete a child's immunizations.
13. See AAP Pediatric Nutrition Handbook (1998) for a discussion of universal and selective screening options. Consider earlier screening for high-risk infants (eg, premature infants and low birth weight infants). See also "Recommendations to Prevent and Control Iron Deficiency in the United States," MMWR. 1998;47 (RR-3):1-29.
14. All menstruating adolescents should be screened annually.
15. Conduct dipstick urinalysis for leukocytes annually for sexually active male and female adolescents.
16. For children at risk of lead exposure consult the AAP statement "Screening for Elevated Blood Lead Levels" (1998). Additionally, screening should be done in accordance with state law where applicable.
17. TB testing per recommendations of the Committee on Infectious Diseases, published in the current edition of Red Book: Report of the Committee on Infectious Diseases. Testing should be done upon recognition of high-risk factors.
18. Cholesterol screening for high-risk patients per AAP statement "Cholesterol in Childhood" (1998). If family history cannot be ascertained and other risk factors are present, screening should be at the discretion of the physician.
19. All sexually active patients should be screened for sexually transmitted diseases (STDs).
20. All sexually active females should have a pelvic examination. A pelvic examination and routine pap smear should be offered as part of preventive health maintenance between the ages of 18 and 21 years.
21. Age-appropriate discussion and counseling should be an integral part of each visit for care per the AAP Guidelines for Health Supervision III (1998).
22. From birth to age 12, refer to the AAP injury prevention program (TIPP) as described in A Guide to Safety Counseling in Office Practice (1994).
23. Violence prevention and management for all patients per AAP statement "The Role of the Pediatrician in Youth Violence Prevention in Clinical Practice and at the Community Level" (1999).
24. Parents and caregivers should be advised to place healthy infants on their backs when putting them to sleep. Side positioning is a reasonable alternative but carries a slightly higher risk of SIDS. Consult the AAP statement "Changing Concepts of Sudden Infant Death Syndrome: Implications for Infant Sleeping Environment and Sleep Position" (2000).
25. Age-appropriate nutrition counseling should be an integral part of each visit per the AAP Handbook of Nutrition (1998).
26. Earlier initial dental examinations may be appropriate for some children. Subsequent examinations as prescribed by dentist.

NB. Special chemical, immunologic, and endocrine testing is usually carried out upon specific indications. Testing other than newborn (eg, inborn errors of metabolism, sickle disease, etc) is discretionary with the physician.

The recommendations in this statement do not indicate an exclusive course of treatment or standard of medical care. Variations, taking into account individual circumstances, may be appropriate. Copyright© 2000 by the American Academy of Pediatrics. No part of this statement may be reproduced in any form or by any means without prior written permission from the American Academy of Pediatrics except for one copy for personal use.

Key:
● = to be performed
★ = to be performed
S = subjective, by history
O = objective, by a standard testing method
←→ = the range during which a service may be provided, with the dot indicating the preferred age.

American Academy of Pediatrics
DEDICATED TO THE HEALTH OF ALL CHILDREN™

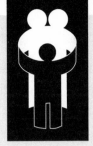

Appendix B.
American Academy of Pediatrics
Publications for Pediatricians and
Parents and Other Caregivers

Books*

Books for Pediatricians

◆ *The Classification of Child and Adolescent Mental Diagnoses in Primary Care: Diagnostic and Statistical Manual for Primary Care (DSM-PC) Child and Adolescent Version,* 1996
This book is a step-by-step guide for assessing and diagnosing mental conditions and making appropriate referrals. Symptom lists for simple, comprehensive diagnoses and the differential diagnosis of mental vs physical and psychosocial problems are included. Use of this book enhances communication with mental health professionals. The book also includes charts, tables, and graphs.

◆ *Handbook of Common Poisonings in Children,* 1994

◆ *Substance Abuse: A Guide for Health Professionals,* 2001

◆ *Pediatric Nutrition Handbook,* 1998; also on CD-ROM

◆ *Injury Prevention and Control for Children and Youth,* 1997

◆ *Care of the Young Athlete,* 2000

Books for Parents

- *Caring for Your Baby and Young Child: Birth to Age 5,* 1998; also in Spanish, 2001
- *Caring for Your School-Age Child: Ages 5 to 12,* 1999
- *Caring for Your Adolescent: Ages 12 to 21,* 1991
- *Guide to Your Child's Symptoms,* 1997
- *Guide to Your Child's Nutrition,* 1999
- *Guide to Your Child's Sleep,* 1999
- *Your Baby's First Year,* 1998

Patient Education Materials for Use in the Pediatric Office*

Parent and Child Guides

- Parent and Child Guides to Pediatric Visits
  Parent and Child guides are available to supplement the *Guidelines for Health Supervision III.* Six age-appropriate parent guides and 3 children's guides give parents and children a list of typical developmental issues for possible discussion with the pediatrician. The guides support the therapeutic alliance between the parent/child and pediatrician and facilitate effective, focused interactions. The guides help share the parents' expectations for the visit and encourage parents to come prepared with questions for the pediatrician.

Vaccines Information Statements

Brochures

- Acne Treatment and Control
- Alcohol: Your Child and Drugs
- Allergies in Children
- Baby Bottle Tooth Decay—How to Prevent It—Fact Sheet
- Baby Walkers Are Very Dangerous!—Fact Sheet
- Bed-wetting
- Better Health and Fitness Through Physical Activity
- Child Care: What's Best for Your Family?
- Child Safety Slips (TIPP)
- Child Sexual Abuse: What It Is and How to Prevent It
- Choking Prevention and First Aid for Infants and Children
- Circumcision: Information for Parents

- Cocaine: Your Child and Drugs
- The Correct Use of Condoms: A Message to Teens
- Deciding to Wait
- Diaper Rash
- Diarrhea and Dehydration
- Discipline and Your Child
- Divorce and Children
- Eating Disorders: What You Should Know About Anorexia and Bulimia
- Environmental Tobacco Smoke: A Danger to Children
- Feeding Kids Right Isn't Always Easy: Tips for Preventing Food Hassles
- For Today's Teens: A Message From Your Pediatrician
- Fun in the Sun: Keep Your Baby Safe
- Gambling: Not a Safe Thrill
- Growing Up Healthy: Fat, Cholesterol, and More
- A Guide to Children's Dental Health
- Health Care for College Students
- Healthy Communication With Your Child
- Important Information for Teens Who Get Headaches
- Infant Sleep Positioning and SIDS—Fact Sheet
- Inhalant Abuse: Your Child and Drugs
- The Internet and Your Family
- Keep Your Family Safe: Fire Safety and Burn Prevention at Home
- Keep Your Family Safe From Firearm Injury
- Know the Facts About HIV and AIDS
- Lead Poisoning: Prevention and Screening
- Learning Disabilities and Children
- Learning Disabilities and Young Adults
- Making the Right Choice: Facts for Teens on Preventing Pregnancy
- Marijuana: Your Child and Drugs
- Newborns: Care of the Uncircumcised Penis—Fact Sheet
- A Parent's Guide to Water Safety
- The Pelvic Exam
- Playground Safety
- Prevent Shaken Baby Syndrome—Fact Sheet
- Protect Your Child From Poison
- Puberty
- Raising Children to Resist Violence: What You Can Do
- The Ratings Game: Choosing Your Child's Entertainment
- Right From the Start: ABCs of Good Nutrition for Young Children
- The Risks of Tobacco Use: A Message to Parents and Teens
- Sex Education: A Bibliography of Educational Materials for Children, Adolescents, and Their Families

- Sibling Relationships
- Single Parenting
- Sleep Problems in Children
- Smoking: Straight Talk for Teens
- Sports and Your Child
- Steroids: Play Safe, Play Fair
- Substance Abuse Prevention: What Every Parent Needs to Know
- Surviving: Coping With Adolescent Depression and Suicide
- Talking With Your Young Child About Sex
- The Teen Driver
- Television and the Family
- Temper Tantrums: A Normal Part of Growing Up
- Testicular/Breast Self-Exam Shower Card
- Thumbs, Fingers, and Pacifiers
- Tips for Parents of Adolescents
- Toilet Training
- Toy Safety
- Treating Jaundice in Healthy Newborns
- 2001 Family Shopping Guide to Car Seats
- Understanding ADHD: Information for Parents About Attention-Deficit/Hyperactivity Disorder
- What's to Eat?: Healthy Foods for Hungry Children
- A Woman's Guide to Breastfeeding
- You and Your Pediatrician
- Your Child and the Environment
- Your Child's Eyes
- Your Child's Growth: Developmental Milestones

Counseling Program*

TIPP®—The Injury Prevention Program
TIPP®—Economy Pack
TIPP®—Age-Related Safety Sheets
TIPP®—Safety Surveys
TIPP®—Bicycle Safety Program
TIPP®—Safety Slips

Policy Statements for Pediatricians*

Committee on Adolescence

- Adolescent Pregnancy—Current Trends and Issues: 1998
- Adolescents and Human Immunodeficiency Virus Infection: The Role of the Pediatrician in Prevention and Intervention (Note: with Committee on Pediatric AIDS)
- Care of Adolescent Parents and Their Children
- Care of the Adolescent Sexual Assault Victim
- Condom Use by Adolescents
- Confidentiality in Adolescent Health Care
- Contraception and Adolescents
- Counseling the Adolescent About Pregnancy Options
- Homosexuality and Adolescence
- Marijuana: A Continuing Concern for Pediatricians
- Sexuality Education for Children and Adolescents (Note: with Committee on Psychosocial Aspects of Child and Family Health)
- Suicide and Suicide Attempts in Adolescents
- The Teenage Driver (Note: with Committee on Injury and Poison Prevention)

Committee on Bioethics

- Appropriate Boundaries in the Pediatrician-Family-Patient Relationship

Committee on Communications

- Children, Adolescents, and Advertising
- Children, Adolescents, and Television
- Impact of Music Lyrics and Music Videos on Children and Youth
- Media Violence
- Sexuality, Contraception, and the Media

Committee on Early Childhood, Adoption, and Dependent Care

- Inappropriate Use of School "Readiness" Tests (Note: with Committee on School Health)
- Pediatrician's Role in Family Support Programs
- Selecting Appropriate Toys for Young Children: The Pediatrician's Role

Committee on Environmental Health

- Environmental Tobacco Smoke: A Hazard to Children
- Ultraviolet Light: A Hazard to Children

Committee on Infectious Diseases

- Immunizations for Native American Children (Note: with Committee on Native American Health)
- Update on Tuberculosis Skin Testing of Children

Committee on Injury and Poison Prevention

- All-Terrain Vehicle Injury Prevention: Two-, Three, and Four-Wheeled Unlicensed Motor Vehicles
- Bicycle Helmets
- Children in Pickup Trucks
- Drowning in Infants, Children, and Adolescents
- Firearm-Related Injuries Affecting the Pediatric Population
- Fireworks-Related Injuries to Children
- Injuries Associated With Infant Walkers
- Injuries Related to "Toy" Firearms
- Lawn Mower-Related Injuries to Children
- Office-Based Counseling for Injury Prevention
- Personal Watercraft Use by Children and Adolescents
- Prevention of Agricultural Injuries Among Children and Adolescents (Note: with Committee on Community Health Services)
- Reducing the Number of Deaths and Injuries From Residential Fires
- Safe Transportation of Newborns at Hospital Discharge
- Skateboard Injuries
- Snowmobiling Hazards
- The Teenage Driver (Note: with Committee on Adolescence)
- Trampolines at Home, School, and Recreational Centers

Committee on Native American Health

- Immunizations for Native American Children (Note: with Committee on Infectious Diseases)

Committee on Nutrition

- Calcium Requirements of Infants, Children, and Adolescents
- Cholesterol in Childhood

Committee on Practice and Ambulatory Medicine

- Eye Examination and Vision Screening in Infants, Children, and Young Adults

Committee on Psychosocial Aspects of Child and Family Health

- Child in Court: A Subject Review
- Guidance for Effective Discipline
- The Pediatrician and Childhood Bereavement
- The Pediatrician and the "New Morbidity"
- Pediatrician's Role in Helping Children and Families Deal With Separation and Divorce
- Prenatal Visit
- Psychosocial Risks of Chronic Health Conditions in Childhood and Adolescence

Committee on School Health

- Corporal Punishment in Schools
- Physical Fitness and Activity in Schools

Committee on Sports Medicine and Fitness

- Adolescents and Anabolic Steroids: A Subject Review
- Amenorrhea in Adolescent Athletes
- Climatic Heat Stress and the Exercising Child and Adolescent
- Horseback Riding and Head Injuries
- Infant Exercise Programs
- Injuries in Youth Soccer: A Subject Review
- In-line Skating Injuries in Children and Adolescents
- Medical Concerns in the Female Athlete
- Organized Sports for Children and Preadolescents (Note: with Committee on School Health)
- Participation in Boxing by Children, Adolescents, and Young Adults
- Promotion of Healthy Weight-control Practices in Young Athletes
- Protective Eyewear for Young Athletes (Note: with the American Academy of Ophthalmology)
- Risk of Injury From Baseball and Softball in Children
- Safety in Youth Ice Hockey: The Effects of Body Checking
- Strength Training by Children and Adolescents
- Swimming Programs for Infants and Toddlers (Note: with the Committee on Injury and Poison Prevention)
- Trampolines at Home, School, and Recreational Centers

Committee on Substance Abuse

- ◆ Alcohol Use and Abuse: A Pediatric Concern
- ◆ Fetal Alcohol Syndrome and Alcohol-Related Neurodevelopmental Disorders
- ◆ Financing of Substance Abuse Treatment for Children and Adolescents
- ◆ Marijuana: A Continuing Concern for Pediatricians
- ◆ Role of Schools in Combatting Substance Abuse
- ◆ Tobacco, Alcohol, and Other Drugs: The Role of the Pediatrician in Prevention and Management of Substance Abuse
- ◆ Tobacco's Toll: Implications for the Pediatrician

Provisional Section on Breastfeeding

- ◆ Breastfeeding and the Use of Human Milk

Task Force on Circumcision

- ◆ Circumcision Policy Statement

Task Force on Infant Sleep Position and Sudden Infant Death Syndrome

- ◆ Changing Concepts of Sudden Infant Death Syndrome: Implications for Infant Sleeping Environment and Sleep Position

Task Force on Newborn and Infant Hearing

- ◆ Newborn and Infant Hearing Loss: Detection and Intervention

Task Force on Infant Sleep Position and SIDS

- ◆ Changing Concepts of Sudden Infant Death Syndrome: Implications for Infant Sleeping Environment and Sleep Position

Task Force on Violence

- ◆ The Role of the Pediatrician in Youth Violence Prevention in Clinical Practice and at the Community Level

---

*This is a selected list of AAP publications most relevant to health supervision. Many other publications, brochures, and statements on illness also are available. New and revised brochures and other publications become available frequently. All current policy statements are available on the AAP Web site (www.aap.org). Parent education materials also are available on CD-ROM. All publications may be ordered from the AAP and a copy of the *AAP Publications Catalog* may be requested at 888/227-1770 between 7:00 am and 5:30 pm central time. Order forms included in the *AAP Publications Catalog* may be faxed to 847/228-1281, ordered from the AAP Web site at www.aap.org (click on BookStore), or mailed to the AAP at 37925 Eagle Way, Chicago, IL 60678-1379 (prepaid orders).

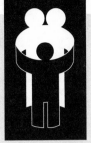

Appendix C.
Parent and Child Guides
to Pediatric Visits

Parents' Guide to Pediatric Visits

Infants Birth to 12 months

Children do best when their parent(s) and their doctors and nurses *work together* to observe them, listen to them, and understand them.

Your first year with your baby is one of the most exciting and important times you will have. It can also be one of the hardest. All babies are different. Perfectly healthy babies have different styles and schedules for eating, sleeping, reacting to noise and touch, and calming themselves when they get upset. Some babies will be very active, and some will seem more calm. Most will enjoy being cuddled, but some will feel more comfortable when they are not held so much. As you watch your baby, you will become the expert on what he or she does more easily, and what your baby needs more help with. Your doctor and nurse can help you with ways to make feeding, sleeping, and discovering the world go well. However, they will need to rely on your report of how your baby does things and what will work best in your household.

As babies grow, they become more regular about when and how long they sleep, when and how they eat, and how they react to you and other important people in their world. You should see signs that your baby hears even soft sounds and sees light and faces. Your baby may turn toward them, watch them, smile at them, and even imitate them. As your baby grows, you will see him or her lifting his/her head, pushing his/her upper body up, and even holding himself/herself up to sit — all so she/he can do even more to see you and the sights and sounds around him/her. If you have a "gut feeling" that there is something wrong or unusual about the way your baby does these things, be sure to talk to your pediatrician about it. Any observation or concern you have is important, and discussing it may help you do even more to help your baby.

It would be helpful if you could take a few minutes to think about what things you would like to discuss during your visit today; the following list is intended to offer a few suggestions.

What are you enjoying most about your baby?

Please put a check (✔) by all areas you would like to discuss:

_____ 1. The baby's health, specific symptoms or concerns

_____ 2. Questions about shots (immunizations) the baby needs

_____ 3. Vision, and how the baby reacts to things she/he sees

_____ 4. Hearing, and how the baby reacts to things she/he hears

_____ 5. How it feels to hold the baby — does she/he feel "tense" or "floppy" or in any way uncomfortable?

_____ 6. When the baby sleeps and for how long

_____ 7. What the baby eats and how often

_____ 8. How active and alert the baby seems to be

_____ 9. Concerns about spoiling the baby

_____ 10. Questions about when the baby might do new things, like sitting or talking

_____ 11. The baby's moods

_____ 12. Questions about bathing or diapering the baby

_____ 13. Questions about child care

_____ 14. Questions about how brothers or sisters interact with the baby

_____ 15. Recovery from pregnancy; questions about family planning or avoiding another pregnancy

_____ 16. Death or illness of a family member

_____ 17. Depression or other psychological problems in a family member

_____ 18. Any accidental injury, trauma, or abuse the child or a parent may have experienced

_____ 19. Other family problems, such as money problems, violence, alcohol, or other drug abuse, conflict between parents, or separation

Are there any *other* concerns you would like to be able to talk about with the doctor or nurse?

Child's name: _____   Today's date: _____

Date of birth: _____

Your name: _____

Your relationship to child: _____

Other people in the household: _____

American Academy of Pediatrics

DEDICATED TO THE HEALTH OF ALL CHILDREN™

HE0221

Parents' Guide to Pediatric Visits

Toddlers 12 to 36 months

Children do best when their parent(s) and their doctors and nurses *work together* to observe them, listen to them, and understand them.

The toddler years are fascinating, exciting, and challenging for parents and children alike. Children are learning to do so many new things so quickly — to walk, to talk, to use the toilet, and to play with other children! They are learning to be more independent and to "have a mind of their own." Children are more and more interested in looking at books and having stories read to them as they advance through the toddler period.

Most parents of toddlers have seen a tantrum, and have had experience with a child who refused to cooperate. Some parents are surprised at how angry they feel under these circumstances. Discussing these issues with family members, friends, or physicians may help parents to think about their preferred approach to discipline.

It would be helpful if you could take a few minutes to think about what things you would like to discuss during your visit today; the following list is intended to offer a few suggestions.

What are you enjoying most about your child at this age?

Please put a check (✔) by all areas you would like to discuss:

_____ 1. The child's health, specific symptoms or concerns

_____ 2. Questions about necessary screening tests or immunizations

_____ 3. Vision or hearing

_____ 4. Appetite or eating patterns

_____ 5. Sleeping patterns and routines, naps

_____ 6. The child's energy or activity level

_____ 7. The child's overall development

_____ 8. The child's ability to speak and be understood

_____ 9. The child's ability to walk, run, climb

_____ 10. Toilet training

_____ 11. Good ways to discipline

_____ 12. Temper tantrums

_____ 13. Fears

_____ 14. How the child behaves with adults

_____ 15. How the child behaves with other children

_____ 16. How the child plays; good ideas for toys and activities

_____ 17. Child care or preschool

_____ 18. The child's relationship with brothers or sisters

_____ 19. Death or illness of a family member

_____ 20. Depression or other psychological problems in a family member

_____ 21. Other family problems, such as money problems, violence, alcohol or other drug abuse, conflicts between parents, or separation

_____ 22. Any trauma or abuse the child may have experienced

_____ 23. Any issues about your own childhood that you think may affect your parenting

Are there any *other* concerns you would like to be able to talk about with the doctor or nurse?

Child's name: _____   Today's date: _____

Date of birth: _____

Your name: _____

Your relationship to child: _____

Other people in the household: _____

American Academy of Pediatrics
DEDICATED TO THE HEALTH OF ALL CHILDREN™

The information contained in this publication should not be used as a substitute for the medical care and advice of your pediatrician. There may be variations in treatment that your pediatrician may recommend based on individual facts and circumstances.

©1997 American Academy of Pediatrics
3-58/Rep0301

HE0222

Parents' Guide to Pediatric Visits

Preschool Children 3 to 5 years old

Children do best when their parent(s) and their doctors and nurses *work together* to observe them, listen to them, and understand them.

The preschool years are busy and exciting times for both parents and children. Children now want to do more and more things for themselves and need help to learn the best ways to dress and feed themselves, take care of bathing and toileting needs, and to explore and play safely. Often they feel "big" enough to try things on their own, but they still need a lot of teaching, supervision, and limits. They are beginning to understand some important learning concepts — numbers, letters, sounds, colors, and shapes. They also are beginning to consider concepts of how to get along — waiting, politeness, sharing, helping, resting. They may be having important experiences of "leaving home" for preschool or recreation activities. There are many differences in how quickly children learn at this age, and their attitudes and interests may be different from those of their brothers, sisters, and friends. They and their parents are learning together about their special skills, interests, and personalities.

It would be helpful if you could take a few minutes to think about what things you would like to discuss during your visit today; the following list is intended to offer a few suggestions.

What are you enjoying most about your child at this age?

Please put a check (✔) by all areas you would like to discuss:

_____ 1. The child's health, specific symptoms or concerns

_____ 2. Questions about necessary screening tests or immunizations

_____ 3. Vision or hearing

_____ 4. Appetite or eating patterns

_____ 5. Sleeping patterns and routines, naps

_____ 6. The child's overall development

_____ 7. The child's ability to speak and be understood

_____ 8. The child's ability to walk, run, and climb

_____ 9. The child's ability to draw, play with blocks and puzzles

_____ 10. The child's energy or activity level

_____ 11. Fears

_____ 12. The child's ability to pay attention to directions or tasks

_____ 13. Toilet training

_____ 14. Sexual behavior or masturbation

_____ 15. Temper tantrums

_____ 16. Good ways to discipline

_____ 17. Child care or preschool arrangements, plans for kindergarten

_____ 18. How the child plays; good ideas for toys and activities

_____ 19. How the child behaves with adults

_____ 20. How the child behaves with other children

_____ 21. The child's relationship with brothers or sisters

_____ 22. Death or illness of a family member

_____ 23. Depression or other psychological problems in a family member

_____ 24. Other family problems, such as money problems, violence, alcohol or other drug abuse, conflicts between parents, or separation

_____ 25. Any trauma or abuse the child may have experienced

_____ 26. Any issues from your childhood that you think may affect your parenting

Are there any *other* concerns you would like to be able to talk about with the doctor or nurse?

Child's name:

Date of birth:

Your name:

Your relationship to child:

Other people in the household:

Today's date:

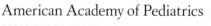

American Academy of Pediatrics

DEDICATED TO THE HEALTH OF ALL CHILDREN™

HE0223

Parents' Guide to Pediatric Visits

School-age Children 6 to 11 years old

Throughout the school years, children are becoming increasingly independent individuals. They are rapidly obtaining new skills, knowledge, and interests. Experiences outside of the home contribute increasingly to their psychological and social growth. During this period, children become increasingly able to make important decisions that influence their health.

The health supervision of school-age children includes attention to their physical, psychological, and social well-being. Health supervision visits provide opportunities to help children gain knowledge about their health and bodies and feel growing responsibility for making healthy decisions. For this reason, it is often helpful for children to be involved directly in discussions during these visits.

It would be helpful if you could take a few minutes to think about what things you would like to discuss during your visit today; the following list is intended to offer a few suggestions.

What are you enjoying most about your child at this age?

Please put a check (✔) by all areas you would like to discuss:

_____ 1. The child's general health, including specific symptoms or concerns

_____ 2. Physical growth and development

_____ 3. Questions about necessary screening tests, immunizations, or the physical examination

_____ 4. Gross- or fine-motor skills

_____ 5. The child's ability to communicate

_____ 6. Bowel and bladder function

_____ 7. Appetite or diet

_____ 8. Sleeping patterns and difficulties

_____ 9. Energy or activity level

_____ 10. Mood (sad, angry, hopeless)

_____ 11. Discipline strategies

_____ 12. School performance or adjustment

_____ 13. School absences

_____ 14. Fears

_____ 15. How the child gets along with other children

_____ 16. How the child interacts with adults

_____ 17. The child's interests and activities

_____ 18. Frequent aches and pains

_____ 19. Questions about sexuality

_____ 20. Annoying habits (like biting nails, sucking thumb)

_____ 21. The child's ability to deal with frustrations

_____ 22. The child's ability to be independent

_____ 23. Attention span

_____ 24. Child care or after-school arrangements

_____ 25. Relationship among family members

_____ 26. Death or illness of a family member

_____ 27. Depression or other psychological difficulties in a family member

_____ 28. Other family stresses (like employment issues, money problems, violence, alcohol or other drug use, conflicts between parents, separation)

_____ 29. Any trauma or abuse the child may have experienced

_____ 30. Any issues from your own childhood that you think might affect your parenting

Are there any *other* concerns you would like to be able to talk about with the doctor or nurse?

Child's name: _____   Today's date: _____

Date of birth: _____

Your name: _____

Your relationship to child: _____

Other people in the household: _____

American Academy of Pediatrics
DEDICATED TO THE HEALTH OF ALL CHILDREN™

Parents' Guide to Pediatric Visits

Younger Adolescents 11 to 15 years old

As children mature, they become much more interested in and capable of assuming responsibility for their own health needs. They show increased concern with their developing body and compare themselves with peers to reassure themselves that they are "normal." Psychological and social independence is increasing, and often teenagers begin to show unwillingness to participate in some family activities. They concentrate instead on peer relationships and social activities. Their social and emotional life can greatly influence their physical health. Risk-taking behaviors are more commonly observed during these years. Early adolescence may be a particularly trying time for both parents and adolescents.

During these years, it becomes appropriate to emphasize the opportunity for adolescent-initiated visits and confidential discussion/ examination without a parent present. It is also important for the parent(s) to speak with the pediatrician alone to communicate your observations and concerns.

What are some of the things that make you especially proud of your adolescent?

Please put a check (✔) by all areas you would like to discuss:

____ 1. Health, specific symptoms or concerns

____ 2. Appetite, eating habits, nutrition

____ 3. Physical growth and development

____ 4. Sexual development, sexual behavior, or sexual orientation

____ 5. Sleeping patterns and routines

____ 6. School performance this year (grades, frequency of absences)

____ 7. Participation in sports

____ 8. Friendships/response to peer pressures

____ 9. Relationships with brothers and sisters

____ 10. Interactions with parent(s)

____ 11. Disciplinary methods, privileges, chores

____ 12. Communicating feelings and concerns

____ 13. Sadness, depression

____ 14. Use of tobacco, alcohol, illicit drugs, or anabolic steroids

____ 15. Family problems, such as money problems, violence, alcohol or other drug abuse, conflicts between parents or separation

____ 16. Death or illness of a family member

____ 17. Any trauma or abuse the adolescent may have experienced

____ 18. Any particular fears

____ 19. Your experience as a teenager and the impact it has on your parenting

Are there any *other* concerns you would like to be able to talk about with the doctor or nurse?

Adolescent's name:	Today's date:
Date of birth:	
Your name:	
Your relationship to adolescent:	
Other people in the household:	

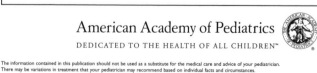

American Academy of Pediatrics
DEDICATED TO THE HEALTH OF ALL CHILDREN™

HE0225

Parents' Guide to Pediatric Visits

Older Adolescents 16 to 21 years old

Adolescents 16 to 21 years of age typically show increasing intellectual, moral, social, and emotional independence. Many teenagers substitute their own or their friends' standards for their family's value system. They may experiment with behaviors that put them at physical, psychological, or social risk. They enter into intimate relationships. Parents are excited and challenged by these developments. Conflicts within the family may occur during this period.

Adolescents do best when their parents and their doctors and nurses respect their autonomy and offer nonjudgmental support and advice. We demonstrate our respect for teenagers by examining them without their parents present and by promising them confidentiality. We want to assure you we will inform you if your adolescent poses a serious risk to himself or herself or to others. We will answer your questions as completely as possible without violating confidentiality. We usually encourage adolescents to discuss issues openly with their families.

It would be helpful if you could take a few minutes to think about what things you would like to discuss during your visit today; the following list is intended to offer a few suggestions.

What are you enjoying most about your adolescent at this age?

Please put a check (✔) by all areas you would like to discuss:

_____ 1. Your adolescent's overall health, or specific symptoms or concerns

_____ 2. Physical growth, development, or stage of puberty

_____ 3. Menstrual patterns or problems

_____ 4. Psychological and social development

_____ 5. Appetite, eating patterns, or nutrition

_____ 6. Sleeping patterns

_____ 7. Emotional outbursts or withdrawal

_____ 8. Evidence of depression or anxiety

_____ 9. Conflicts in the family

_____ 10. Family problems, such as money problems, violence, alcohol or other drug use, separation or divorce

_____ 11. School attendance or performance

_____ 12. Stealing or taking things that do not belong to him/her

_____ 13. Sports participation

_____ 14. Fears

_____ 15. Friends and peer group

_____ 16. Angry or irritable moods

_____ 17. Smoking

_____ 18. Alcohol use

_____ 19. Use of other drugs

_____ 20. Sexual orientation

_____ 21. Sexual activity

_____ 22. Unsafe activities or practices

_____ 23. Immunizations required at this age

_____ 24. Special screening tests

_____ 25. Any trauma or abuse

_____ 26. Planning for job or further education

Are there any *other* concerns you would like to be able to talk about with the doctor or nurse?

Adolescent's name:

Date of birth:

Your name:

Your relationship to adolescent:

Other people in the household:

Today's date:

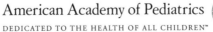

American Academy of Pediatrics
DEDICATED TO THE HEALTH OF ALL CHILDREN™

Child's Guide to Pediatric Visits

School-age Children 6 to 11 years old

In the past year or two you have learned a lot of new information and skills, both at home and at school. You can now do more on your own and you probably are involved in a lot of activities. You may have discovered new people and new experiences that are important to you.

You are also becoming able to make good decisions about your health and safety. For example, you can remember to *wear your helmet* when you are riding your bike, *buckle up your seat belts* anytime you ride in a car, *brush your teeth, eat nutritious foods, and avoid alcohol and tobacco use.* You can also let your doctor know how you are feeling, and ask any questions you have about your health, your friends, school, your family, or experiences you have had.

It would be helpful if you could take a few minutes now to think about what things you would like to discuss during your visit with your doctor today. The following list is intended to give you a few suggestions.

What is one thing you are proud of about yourself?

Please put a check (✔) by all areas you would like to discuss:

_____ 1. Your general health, or particular symptoms or concerns

_____ 2. Your physical growth

_____ 3. Questions about any aspect of your medical care or what will happen at today's visit

_____ 4. Your school work

_____ 5. Sports and other activities

_____ 6. Urinating or having bowel movements

_____ 7. Your appetite or diet

_____ 8. Your sleeping

_____ 9. Your energy or activity level

_____ 10. How you get along with other children

_____ 11. How you get along with your brothers and sisters

_____ 12. How you get along with your mother and father

_____ 13. Any aches and pains you have frequently

_____ 14. Any things you have been worrying about

_____ 15. Any injuries you have had

_____ 16. The effects of tobacco, alcohol, and other drugs of abuse

Are there any *other* concerns you would like to be able to talk about with the doctor or nurse?

Your name: Today's date:

Date of birth:

Parent(s)' name(s):

Other people in the household:

American Academy of Pediatrics
DEDICATED TO THE HEALTH OF ALL CHILDREN™

HE0228

Child's Guide to Pediatric Visits

Younger Adolescents 11 to 15 years old

As an adolescent, during your visits to the pediatrician, you will have the opportunity to meet with the doctor or nurse to talk confidentially about issues that concern you.

It is common for young adolescents to have concerns about their rapid physical growth and sexual development (puberty). It is important to feel accepted among your peers over standards for dress, recreation, behavior, and values. Adolescents experiment with many risk-taking behaviors. Conflicts with parents over issues of independence are common.

During these visits, you may bring up for discussion anything that concerns you. Some issues that commonly worry children and teenagers are listed below. Be assured that confidentiality will be maintained unless the doctor or nurse is concerned that you are going to hurt yourself or someone else.

What are some of the things that make you feel proud of yourself?

Please put a check (✔) by all areas you would like to discuss:

____ 1. Any health issue, specific symptom or concern

____ 2. Your eating or weight

____ 3. Sleeping pattern and routines

____ 4. Bowel and urine elimination

____ 5. For girls — menstrual history (regularity/length of period/pain) For boys — "nocturnal emissions" (wet dreams)

____ 6. School grades

____ 7. Any problems with school

____ 8. Sports, hobbies, or other activities

____ 9. Your friends

____ 10. Interactions with your brothers and sisters

____ 11. Interactions with your parent(s)

____ 12. Responsibilities at home, chores, household rules

____ 13. Feelings of sadness, mood changes

____ 14. Worrying a lot

____ 15. Trouble concentrating

____ 16. Frequent aches and pains

____ 17. Feeling angry or hopeless

____ 18. Taking unnecessary risks

____ 19. Use of tobacco or alcohol

____ 20. Other drugs or anabolic steroids

____ 21. Sexual activity, contraceptives, sexually transmitted diseases

____ 22. Your sexual orientation

____ 23. Fears

____ 24. Family problems, such as money problems, violence, alcohol or other drug abuse, conflicts between parents or separation

____ 25. Death or illness of a family member

____ 26. Any trauma or abuse you have experienced

Are there any *other* concerns you would like to be able to talk about with the doctor or nurse?

Your name:

Date of birth:

Parent(s)' name(s):

Other people in the household:

Today's date:

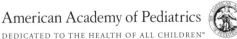

American Academy of Pediatrics
DEDICATED TO THE HEALTH OF ALL CHILDREN™

Child's Guide to Pediatric Visits

Older Adolescents 16 to 21 years old

As an older adolescent, we would like to acknowledge your individuality by examining you without your parents present. We promise you confidentiality. We will inform your parents about our discussions only if you are doing or thinking things that pose a serious risk to yourself or to others. We may encourage you to discuss some issues openly with your family. We can brainstorm with you about how to do this.

During these years, teens typically show increasing intellectual, moral, social, and emotional independence. You may have substituted your own or your friends' standards for your family's value system. You may be experimenting with behaviors that put you at physical, psychological, or social risk. Many teens develop intimate relationships during this age and begin thinking about sexual activity. The possibility of conflict within the family increases in this period.

It would be helpful if you could take a few minutes to think about what things you would like to discuss during your visit today; the following list is intended to offer a few suggestions.

What are you happy about or proud of in yourself?

Please put a check (✔) by all areas you would like to discuss:

_____ 1. Your overall health, or specific symptoms or concerns

_____ 2. Your physical development or stage of puberty

_____ 3. Menstrual patterns or problems

_____ 4. Your social and emotional needs

_____ 5. Appetite, eating patterns, or nutrition

_____ 6. Your sleeping patterns

_____ 7. Emotional problems, such as depression or anxiety

_____ 8. Family problems, such as money problems, violence, alcohol or other drug use, separation or divorce

_____ 9. Communication patterns in your family

_____ 10. Problems with your parents

_____ 11. Any problems at school

_____ 12. Your school performance

_____ 13. Preparation for future education or job

_____ 14. Sports participation

_____ 15. Your friends and peer group

_____ 16. Angry or irritable moods

_____ 17. Smoking

_____ 18. Fears or anxiety you may have

_____ 19. Alcohol use

_____ 20. Use of other drugs

_____ 21. Your sexual orientation

_____ 22. Your sexual activity

_____ 23. Unsafe, high-risk activities or practices

_____ 24. Immunizations required at this age

_____ 25. Special screening tests

_____ 26. Any abuse or trauma you have experienced

_____ 27. Planning for job or further education

Are there any *other* concerns you would like to be able to talk about with the doctor or nurse?

Your name: _____   Today's date: _____

Date of birth: _____

Parent(s)' name(s): _____

Other people in the household: _____

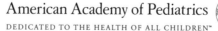

American Academy of Pediatrics
DEDICATED TO THE HEALTH OF ALL CHILDREN™

HE0230

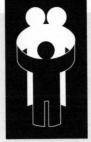

Appendix D.
Recommended
Childhood Immunization
Schedule

Recommended Childhood Immunization Schedule
United States, January – December 2001*

Vaccines[1] are listed under routinely recommended ages. Bars indicate range of recommended ages. Any dose not given at the recommended age should be given as a "catch-up" immunization at any subsequent visit when indicated and feasible. Ovals indicate vaccines to be given if previously recommended doses were missed or given earlier than the recommended minimum age.

Age ▶ Vaccine ▼	Birth	1 mo	2 mos	4 mos	6 mos	12 mos	15 mos	18 mos	24 mos	4-6 yrs	11-12 yrs	14-18 yrs
Hepatitis B[2]		Hep B #1	Hep B #2			Hep B #3					Hep B[2]	
Diphtheria, Tetanus, Pertussis[3]			DTaP	DTaP	DTaP			DTaP[3]		DTaP	Td	Td
H. influenzae type b[4]			Hib	Hib	Hib	Hib						
Inactivated Polio[5]			IPV	IPV		IPV[5]				IPV[5]		
Pneumococcal Conjugate[6]			PCV	PCV	PCV	PCV						
Measles, Mumps, Rubella[7]						MMR				MMR[7]	MMR[7]	
Varicella[8]						Var					Var[8]	
Hepatitis A[9]									Hep A-in selected areas[9]			

Approved by the Advisory Committee on Immunization Practices (ACIP), the American Academy of Pediatrics (AAP), and the American Academy of Family Physicians (AAFP).

*The immunization schedule is updated annually. Please access the current schedule at http://www.aap.org/family/parents/immunize.htm.

1. This schedule indicates the recommended ages for routine administration of currently licensed childhood vaccines, as of 11/1/00, for children through 18 years of age. Additional vaccines may be licensed and recommended during the year. Licensed combination vaccines may be used whenever any components of the combination are indicated and its other components are not contraindicated. Providers should consult the manufacturers' package inserts for detailed recommendations.

2. **Infants born to HBsAg-negative mothers** should receive the 1st dose of hepatitis B (Hep B) vaccine by age 2 months. The 2nd dose should be at least one month after the 1st dose. The 3rd dose should be administered at least 4 months after the 1st dose and at least 2 months after the 2nd dose, but not before 6 months of age for infants.

Infants born to HBsAg-positive mothers should receive hepatitis B vaccine and 0.5 mL hepatitis B immune globulin (HBIG) within 12 hours of birth at separate sites The 2nd dose is recommended at 1-2 months of age and the 3rd dose at 6 months of age.

Infants born to mothers whose HBsAg status is unknown should receive hepatitis B vaccine within 12 hours of birth. Maternal blood should be drawn at the time of delivery to determine the mother's HBsAg status; if the HBsAg test is positive, the infant should receive HBIG as soon as possible (no later than 1 week of age).

All children and adolescents who have not been immunized against hepatitis B should begin the series during any visit. Special efforts should be made to immunize children who were born in or whose parents were born in areas of the world with moderate or high endemicity of hepatitis B virus infection.

3. The 4th dose of DTaP (diphtheria and tetanus toxoids and acellular pertussis vaccine) may be administered as early as 12 months of age, provided 6 months have elapsed since the 3rd dose and the child is unlikely to return at age 15-18 months. Td (tetanus and diphtheria toxoids) is recommended at 11-12 years of age if at least 5 years have elapsed since the last dose of DTP, DTaP or DT. Subsequent routine Td boosters are recommended every 10 years.

4. Three *Haemophilus influenzae* type b (Hib) conjugate vaccines are licensed for infant use. If PRP-OMP (PedvaxHIB® or ComVax® [Merck]) is administered at 2 and 4 months of age, a dose at 6 months is not required. Because clinical studies in infants have demonstrated that using some combination products may induce a lower immune response to the Hib vaccine component, DTaP/Hib combination products should not be used for primary immunization in infants at 2, 4 or 6 months of age, unless FDA-approved for these ages.

5. An all-IPV schedule is recommended for routine childhood polio vaccination in the United States. All children should receive four doses of IPV at 2 months, 4 months, 6-18 months, and 4-6 years of age. Oral polio vaccine (OPV) should be used only in selected circumstances. (See *MMWR Morb Mortal Wkly Rep* May 19, 2000/49(RR-5):1-22).

6. The heptavalent conjugate pneumococcal vaccine (PCV) is recommended for all children 2-23 months of age. It also is recommended for certain children 24-59 months of age. (See *MMWR Morb Mortal Wkly Rep* Oct. 6, 2000/49(RR-9):1-35).

7. The 2nd dose of measles, mumps, and rubella (MMR) vaccine is recommended routinely at 4-6 years of age but may be administered during any visit, provided at least 4 weeks have elapsed since receipt of the 1st dose and that both doses are administered beginning at or after 12 months of age. Those who have not previously received the second dose should complete the schedule by the 11-12 year old visit.

8. Varicella (Var) vaccine is recommended at any visit on or after the first birthday for susceptible children, i.e. those who lack a reliable history of chickenpox (as judged by a health care provider) and who have not been immunized. Susceptible persons 13 years of age or older should receive 2 doses, given at least 4 weeks apart.

9. Hepatitis A (Hep A) is shaded to indicate its recommended use in selected states and/or regions, and for certain high risk groups; consult your local public health authority. (See *MMWR Morb Mortal Wkly Rep* Oct. 1, 1999/48(RR-12); 1-37).

For additional information about the vaccines listed above, please visit the National Immunization Program Home Page at www.cdc.gov/nip or call the National Immunization Hotline at 800-232-2522 (English) or 800-232-0233 (Spanish).

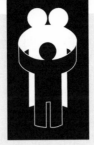

Appendix E.
Preparing Parents for
Emergency Medical Services:
A Parents' Guide

When your child needs emergency medical services

It is rare for children to become seriously ill with no warning. Based on your child's symptoms, you should usually contact your child's pediatrician for advice. Timely treatment of symptoms can prevent an illness from getting worse or turning into an emergency.

What is a true emergency?

A true emergency is when you believe a severe injury or illness is threatening your child's life or may cause permanent harm. In these cases, a child needs emergency medical treatment right away.

Discuss with your child's pediatrician in advance what you should do in case of a true emergency.

Many true emergencies involve sudden injuries. These injuries are often caused by the following:
- ◆ Bicycle or car crashes, falls, or other violent impacts
- ◆ Poisoning
- ◆ Burns or smoke inhalation
- ◆ Choking
- ◆ Near drowning
- ◆ Firearms or other weapons
- ◆ Electric shocks

Other true emergencies can result from either medical illnesses or injuries. You can often tell that these emergencies are happening if you observe your child showing any of the following:

♦ Acting strangely or becoming more withdrawn and less alert
♦ Increasing trouble with breathing
♦ Bleeding that does not stop
♦ Skin or lips that look blue or purple (or gray for darker-skinned children)
♦ Rhythmical jerking and loss of consciousness (a seizure)
♦ Unconsciousness
♦ Very loose or knocked-out teeth, or other major mouth or facial injuries
♦ Increasing or severe persistent pain
♦ A cut or burn that is large or deep
♦ Any loss of consciousness, confusion, a bad headache, or vomiting several times **after a head injury**
♦ Decreasing responsiveness when you talk to your child

Call your child's pediatrician or poison control center at once if your child has swallowed a suspected poison or another person's medication, even if your child has no signs or symptoms.

Always call for help if you are concerned that your child's life may be in danger or that your child is seriously hurt.

In case of a true emergency

♦ Stay calm.
♦ If it is needed and you know how, start rescue breathing or CPR (cardio-pulmonary resuscitation).
♦ If you need immediate help, call "911." If you do not have "911" service in your area, call your local emergency ambulance service or county emergency medical service. Otherwise, call your child's pediatrician's office and state clearly that you have an emergency.
♦ If there is bleeding, apply continuous pressure to the site with a clean cloth.
♦ If your child is having a seizure, place her on a carpeted floor with her head turned to the side, and stay with your child until help arrives.

After you arrive at the emergency department, make sure you tell the emergency staff the name of your child's pediatrician who can work closely with the emergency department and can provide them with additional information about your child. Bring any medication your child is taking and his immunization record with you to the hospital. Also bring any suspected poisons or other medications your child might have taken.

Important Emergency Telephone Numbers

Keep the following telephone numbers handy by taping them on or near your telephone:

- Your home telephone and address
- Your child's pediatrician
- Emergency medical services (ambulance) (911 in most areas)
- Police (911 in most areas)
- Fire department (911 in most areas)
- Poison control center
- Hospital
- Dentist

It is important that baby-sitters know where to find emergency telephone numbers. If you have "911" service in your area, make sure they know to dial "911" in case of an emergency. Be sure your baby-sitter knows your home address and telephone number, since an emergency operator would ask for this information. Always leave your baby-sitter the telephone number and address where you can be located.

Remember, for any emergency always call your child's pediatrician or EMS. If your child is seriously ill or injured, it may be safer for your child to be transported by emergency medical services.

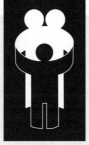

Appendix F.
Recommendations for
Tuberculosis Testing

◆ All children need routine health care evaluations that include assessment of their risk of exposure to tuberculosis. Only children deemed to have increased risk of exposure to persons with tuberculosis should be considered for tuberculin (Mantoux) skin testing. The frequency of such skin testing should be according to the degree of risk of acquiring tuberculous infection as detailed in Table 1.

◆ Routine tuberculin skin testing of children with no risk factors residing in low-prevalence communities is not indicated.

◆ Children who have no risk factors but who reside in high-prevalence regions and children whose histories for risk factors are incomplete or unreliable should be considered for tuberculin (Mantoux) skin testing at 4 to 6 and 11 to 16 years of age. The decision to test should be based on the local epidemiology of tuberculosis in conjunction with advice from regional tuberculosis control officials.

◆ Family investigation is indicated whenever a tuberculin skin test result of a parent converts from negative to positive (indicating recent infection). Children of health care workers are not at increased risk of acquiring tuberculous infection unless the workers' tuberculin skin test results convert to positive or the workers have diagnoses of tuberculous disease.

◆ Children with human immunodeficiency virus (HIV) infection or disease should receive annual tuberculin skin testing (5 tuberculin units, Mantoux).

◆ The skin test interpretation guidelines for indurations of 5, 10, and 15 mm in diameter (Table 2) remain appropriate for decisions regarding contact investigations, tuberculosis control measures, and preventive therapy.

Table 1.
Revised Tuberculin Skin Test Recommendations*

Children for whom immediate skin testing is indicated

* Contacts of persons with confirmed or suspected infectious tuberculosis (contact investigation); this includes children identified as contacts of family members or associates in jail or prison in the last 5 y
* Children with radiographic or clinical findings suggesting tuberculosis
* Children immigrating from endemic countries (eg, Asia, Middle East, Africa, Latin America)
* Children with travel histories to endemic countries and/or significant contact with indigenous persons from such countries

Children who should be tested annually for tuberculosis†

* Children infected with HIV
* Incarcerated adolescents

Children who should be tested every 2–3 y†

* Children exposed to the following individuals: HIV infected, homeless, residents of nursing homes, institutionalized adolescents or adults, users of illicit drugs, incarcerated adolescents or adults, and migrant farmworkers; this would include foster children with exposure to adults in the above high-risk groups

Children who should be considered for tuberculin skin testing at ages 4–6 and 11–16 y

* Children whose parents immigrated (with unknown tuberculin skin test status) from regions of the world with high prevalence of tuberculosis; continued potential exposure by travel to the endemic areas and/or household contact with persons from the endemic areas (with unknown tuberculin skin test status) should be an indication for repeat tuberculin skin testing
* Children without specific risk factors who reside in high-prevalence areas; in general, a high-risk neighborhood or community does not mean an entire city is at high risk; it is recognized that rates in any area of the city may vary by neighborhood, or even from block to block; physicians should be aware of these patterns in determining the likelihood of exposure; public health officials or local tuberculosis experts should help clinicians identify areas that have appreciable tuberculosis rates

Risk for progression to disease

* Children with other medical risk factors, including diabetes mellitus, chronic renal failure, malnutrition, and congenital or acquired immunodeficiencies deserve special consideration; without recent exposure, these persons are not at increased risk of acquiring tuberculous infection; underlying immunodeficiencies associated with these conditions theoretically would enhance the possibility for progression to severe disease; initial histories of potential exposure to tuberculosis should be included on all of these patients; if these histories or local epidemiologic factors suggest a possibility of exposure, immediate and periodic tuberculin skin testing should be considered in these patients; an initial Mantoux tuberculin skin test should be performed before initiation of immunosuppressive therapy in any child with an underlying condition that necessitates immunosuppressive therapy

*BCG immunization is not a contraindication to tuberculin skin testing.
†Initial tuberculin skin testing initiated at the time of diagnosis or circumstance.

Table 2.
Definition of a Positive Mantoux Skin Test (5 Tuberculin Units of Purified Protein Derivative) in Children*

Reaction ≥5 mm
- Children in close contact with known or suspected infectious cases of tuberculosis
  - Households with active or previously active cases if treatment cannot be verified as adequate before exposure, treatment was initiated after the child's contact, or reactivation is suspected

- Children suspected to have tuberculosis disease
  - Chest roentgenogram consistent with active or previously active tuberculosis
  - Clinical evidence of tuberculosis[†]

- Children receiving immunosuppressive therapy[‡] or with immunosuppressive conditions, including HIV infection

Reaction ≥10 mm
- Children at increased risk of dissemination
  - Young age (<4 y)
  - Other medical risk factors, including diabetes mellitus, chronic renal failure, or malnutrition

- Children with increased environmental exposure
  - Born, or whose parents were born, in high-prevalence regions of the world
  - Frequently exposed to adults who are HIV infected, homeless, users of illicit drugs, medically indigent city dwellers, residents of nursing homes, incarcerated or institutionalized persons, and migrant farmworkers

- Travel and exposure to high-prevalence regions of the world

Reaction ≥15 mm
- Children ≥4 y of age without any risk factors

*The recommendations should be considered regardless of previous BCG administration.

†Evidence on physical examinations or laboratory assessment that would include tuberculosis in the working diagnosis (ie, meningitis).

‡Including immunosuppressive doses of corticosteroids.

Appendix F is from the American Academy of Pediatrics, Committee on Infectious Diseases. Update on tuberculosis skin testing of children. *Pediatrics.* 1996;97:282–284.

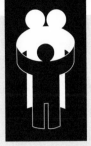

Appendix G.
Lead Toxicity Screening

Screening should begin at 9 to 12 months and be resumed at about 24 months. If universal screening is recommended for the community, follow the community standards (check with public health authority). When targeted screening is recommended, assess each child for risk and screen as necessary. Assess periodically between 6 months and 6 years of age using community-specific risk-assessment questions. (See the AAP policy statement, Screening for Elevated Blood Lead Levels.)

Questions to assess risk status for lead poisoning.

◆ Does your child spend time in buildings built before 1950 with peeling or chipping paint, including day care centers, preschools, or the homes of baby-sitters or relatives?

◆ Does your child live in or regularly visit buildings built before 1960 with recent, ongoing, or planned renovation or remodeling?

◆ Does your child have a brother or sister, housemate, or playmate being followed up or treated for lead poisoning?

◆ Does your child frequently come in contact with an adult whose job or hobby involves exposure to lead, such as construction, welding, pottery, or other trades?

◆ Does your child live near an active lead smelter, battery recycling plant, or other industry likely to release lead?

◆ Has your child been given home remedies (azarcon, greta, pay looah)?

◆ Has your child lived outside the United States?

◆ If your home was built before 1978, has it been remodeled recently or do you have plans to remodel it?

◆ Do you live within 1 block of a major highway or busy street?

♦ Do you use hot tap water for cooking or drinking?

♦ Does your family use pottery or ceramics for cooking, eating, or drinking?

♦ Have you seen your child eat paint chips, soil, or dirt?

♦ Have you been told your child has low iron?

♦ Does your house have mini-blinds manufactured outside the United States before 1996?

If the answer to any of these questions is YES, the child is considered to be at risk of excessive lead exposure and should be screened with a blood lead test

TABLE 1.   A Basic Personal-Risk Questionnaire*

____Yes	____No	1. Does your child live in or regularly visit a house or child care facility built before 1950?
____Yes	____No	2. Does your child live in or regularly visit a house or child care facility built before 1978 that is being or has recently been renovated or remodeled (within the last 6 months)?
____Yes	____No	3. Does your child have a sibling or playmate who has or did have lead poisoning?

* Adapted from the Centers for Disease Control and Prevention.   The state or local health department may recommend alternative or additional questions based on local conditions. If the answers to the questions are "no," a screening test is not required, although the provider should explain why the questions were asked to reinforce anticipatory guidance. If the answer to either question is "yes" or "not sure," a screening test should be considered.

TABLE 3.   Recommended Follow-up Services, According to Diagnostic BLL

BLL (µg/dL)	Action
<10	No action required

10–14	Obtain a confirmatory venous BLL within 1 month; if still within this range,
	    Provide education to decrease blood lead exposure
	    Repeat BLL test within 3 months

15–19	Obtain a confirmatory venous BLL within 1 month; if still within this range,
	    Take a careful environmental history
	    Provide education to decrease blood lead exposure and to decrease lead absorption
	    Repeat BLL test within 2 months

20–44	Obtain a confirmatory venous BLL within 1 week; if still within this range,
	    Conduct a complete medical history (including an environmental evaluation and nutritional assessment) and physical examination
	    Provide education to decrease blood lead exposure and to decrease lead absorption
	    Either refer the patient to the local health department or provide case management that should include a detailed environmental investigation with lead hazard reduction and appropriate referrals for support services
	    If BLL is >25 µg/dL, consider chelation (not currently recommended for BLLs >45 µg/dL), after consultation with clinicians experienced in lead toxicity treatment

45–69	Obtain a confirmatory venous BLL within 2 days; if still within this range,
	    Conduct a complete medical history (including an environmental evaluation and nutritional assessment) and a physical examination
	    Provide education to decrease blood lead exposure and to decrease lead absorption
	    Either refer the patient to the local health department or provide case management that should include a detailed environmental investigation with lead hazard reduction and appropriate referrals for support services
	    Begin chelation therapy in consultation with clinicians experienced in lead toxicity therapy

70	Hospitalize the patient and begin medical treatment immediately in consultation with clinicians experienced in lead toxicity therapy
	    Obtain a confirmatory BLL immediately
	    The rest of the management should be as noted for management of children with BLLs between 45 and 69 µg/dL

TABLE 4. Risk Factors for Lead Exposure and Prevention Strategies

Risk Factor	Prevention Strategy
Environmental	
Paint	Identify and abate
Dust	Wet mop, frequent handwashing
Soil	Restrict play in area, ground cover, frequent handwashing
Drinking water	2-minute flush of morning water; use of cold water for cooking, drinking
Folk remedies	Avoid use
Old ceramic or pewter cookware, old urns/kettles	Avoid use
Some imported cosmetics, toys, crayons	Avoid use
Parental occupations	Remove work clothing at work
Hobbies	Proper use, storage, and ventilation
Home renovation	Proper containment, ventilation
Buying or renting a new home	Inquire about lead hazards
Host	
Hand-to-mouth activity (or pica)	Frequent handwashing
Inadequate nutrition	High iron and calcium, low-fat diet; frequent small meals
Developmental disabilities	Frequent screening

Tables 1, 3, and 4 from the American Academy of Pediatrics, Committee on Environmental Health. Screening for elevated blood lead levels. *Pediatrics.* 1998;101:1072–1078.